NEUROSCIENCE RESEARCH PROGRESS

UNLOCKING ERIK

A FREEDOM JOURNEY TO RESTORE THE SPEECH OF THOSE WITH LOCKED-IN SYNDROME

NEUROSCIENCE RESEARCH PROGRESS

Additional books and e-books in this series can be found on Nova's website under the Series tab.

NEUROSCIENCE RESEARCH PROGRESS

UNLOCKING ERIK

A FREEDOM JOURNEY TO RESTORE THE SPEECH OF THOSE WITH LOCKED-IN SYNDROME

PHILIP R. KENNEDY, MD, PhD

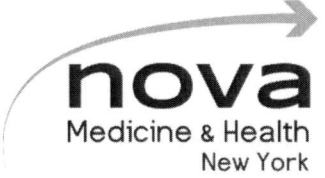

Medicine & Health
New York

Copyright © 2020 by Nova Science Publishers, Inc.

All rights reserved. No part of this book may be reproduced, stored in a retrieval system or transmitted in any form or by any means: electronic, electrostatic, magnetic, tape, mechanical photocopying, recording or otherwise without the written permission of the Publisher.

We have partnered with Copyright Clearance Center to make it easy for you to obtain permissions to reuse content from this publication. Simply navigate to this publication's page on Nova's website and locate the "Get Permission" button below the title description. This button is linked directly to the title's permission page on copyright.com. Alternatively, you can visit copyright.com and search by title, ISBN, or ISSN.

For further questions about using the service on copyright.com, please contact:
Copyright Clearance Center
Phone: +1-(978) 750-8400   Fax: +1-(978) 750-4470   E-mail: info@copyright.com

NOTICE TO THE READER

The Publisher has taken reasonable care in the preparation of this book, but makes no expressed or implied warranty of any kind and assumes no responsibility for any errors or omissions. No liability is assumed for incidental or consequential damages in connection with or arising out of information contained in this book. The Publisher shall not be liable for any special, consequential, or exemplary damages resulting, in whole or in part, from the readers' use of, or reliance upon, this material. Any parts of this book based on government reports are so indicated and copyright is claimed for those parts to the extent applicable to compilations of such works.

Independent verification should be sought for any data, advice or recommendations contained in this book. In addition, no responsibility is assumed by the Publisher for any injury and/or damage to persons or property arising from any methods, products, instructions, ideas or otherwise contained in this publication.

This publication is designed to provide accurate and authoritative information with regard to the subject matter covered herein. It is sold with the clear understanding that the Publisher is not engaged in rendering legal or any other professional services. If legal or any other expert assistance is required, the services of a competent person should be sought. FROM A DECLARATION OF PARTICIPANTS JOINTLY ADOPTED BY A COMMITTEE OF THE AMERICAN BAR ASSOCIATION AND A COMMITTEE OF PUBLISHERS.

Additional color graphics may be available in the e-book version of this book.

Library of Congress Cataloging-in-Publication Data

ISBN: 978-1-53617-455-7
Library of Congress Control Number: 2020931697

Published by Nova Science Publishers, Inc. † New York

"This book has come at an important time in the evolution of the brain machine interface ... *Unlocking Erik* tells the story from the human side – both in terms of Erik himself as the subject, and Dr. Kennedy as the pioneer. It is a journey of quiet and slow discovery, and has taken courage and risk from all sides."

-- Prof. Alexander Green

-- Neurosurgeon, University of Oxford, England.

"With Dr. Kennedy widely regarded as one of the pioneers of this technology, he is uniquely placed to discuss the far-reaching consequences and ramifications of BCI, and this certainly helped attract the funding we needed to begin production of the documentary that tracks early breakthroughs in the field."

--David Burke,

--Dot-television, Ireland

"Finally, with all the excitement of machine learning, we shouldn't forget that we are talking about connecting to a neural network with more capabilities and far more creativity than anything that Google has made – the human brain! So let's try to not forget the brain's ability to learn."

-- Andrew Jackson

-- Professor of Neural Interfaces, University of Newcastle, U.K.

"Phil is a friend, mentor, lunatic, philanthropist, son of the universe and a consummate neuroscientist...I think anyone would agree that the fathers of modern intraoperative neuromodulatory brain surgery in Belize are Dr. Kennedy, the late Roy Bakay MD., and myself. I heartily welcome other Philip Kennedy's and Roy Bakay's to help the scientific world grow neuroscience, neurology, neuropsychiatry and neurosurgery for the benefit of all mankind."

-- Joel Cervantes
Belize Medical Center, Belize City, Belize

"We know that neurons involved in internal "thinking" are also clearly controllable. As explored in Phil Kennedy's study of Erik, the neurons involved in generating speech are a particularly important group of volitionally controllable neurons for speech prostheses."

--Eberhard Fetz
Center for Neurotechnology, Seattle, Washington, USA

"This book tells a remarkable story. There is a group of patients rendered unable to communicate by a brutal medical misfortune. There is a new therapy involving special equipment... and there is the physician who manages their care... Dr. Kennedy has achieved remarkable success with his brain machine inter-faces. He remains focused on the tremendous value of restoring speech to patients who are trapped inside their own bodies..."

--Thomas Wichmann
Department of Neurology, Emory University, Atlanta, Georgia, USA.

Dedicated to all those who are locked-in and all those who will become locked-in.

CONTENTS

Foreword	Pioneers in the Ever-Expanding Field of Brain to Computer Interfacing *Alexander Green*	xiii
Preface	Decades of Opening the Door to the Mind	xvii
Acknowledgments		xxv
Part 1	**Erik's Journey**	**1**
Chapter 1	Breaking the Sound Barrier	3
Chapter 2	Some Superheroes Only Fly Inside	15
Chapter 3	Coding and Decoding Erik's Inner Dialogue	21
Chapter 4	Believing in the Magic, Counting on the Science	27
Chapter 5	Unexpected Delays and Eureka Moments	33
Chapter 6	The Place Where "I" Exists	39
Chapter 7	Deep Presence: Understanding the Here and Now	45
Chapter 8	The Uncharted Waters of Research: 'Here there be Dragons'!	53

Chapter 9	Conversations between Eddie Ramsey and Phil Kennedy on June 3rd and 19th, 2019	59
Part 2	**The Science behind Unlocking Erik**	**85**
Chapter 10	Introduction: "The Inconvenient Details of Locked-In Syndrome"	87
Chapter 11	Erik's Injury	95
Chapter 12	Meeting Dr. Kennedy	97
Chapter 13	The Implant Surgery	101
Chapter 14	Recording from Erik	105
Chapter 15	Using Single Units to Say "Da, Da"	109
Chapter 16	Decoding 22 to 24 of 39 Phones	111
Chapter 17	Moving from Vowel to Vowel	113
Chapter 18	The Effects of Emotion on Firing Rates	117
Chapter 19	Music Relates to Firing Rates	121
Chapter 20	Conditioning Single Units Nine Years after Implantation	123
Chapter 21	Limitations of Erik's Recordings	125
Chapter 22	Phil's Implantation Surgery	127
Chapter 23	Sensory and Motor Relationships	129
Chapter 24	Decoding Most Phones	131
Chapter 25	Decoding Audible and Silent Speech	135
Chapter 26	The Future Direction: Ready to Implant Locked-In People More Successfully?	141
Chapter 27	Why Not Use Other Electrodes and Systems?	143
Chapter 28	The Future Is Almost Here	147

Chapter 29	Scientific Commentaries	**153**
Afterword		**197**
	David Burke	
References		**205**
About the Author		**209**
Index		**211**

Foreword: Pioneers in the Ever-Expanding Field of Brain to Computer Interfacing

I first met Professor Philip Kennedy at the 'Neural Interfaces Conference' in Salt Lake City in 2013. He was quietly standing next to his scientific poster detailing almost 20 years of his research into development of a prosthesis for human speech. Kennedy was modest about his achievements and extremely polite, yet at the same time, I could sense a great enthusiasm, indeed a passion for his work.

His presentation was perhaps a little understated. Most professors leave the poster to their juniors to present. However, when we got talking, I soon realised why he had come to present the work himself. His poster concentrated on some of the technical aspects of his human brain Electrode – trying to get cells from the brain to 'grow' into the Electrodes to keep them working – this has, to date, been one of the problems with the 'Utah arrays' (Electrodes that are an array of pins) that have been implanted onto the motor cortex. These Electrodes generate 'gliosis' or scarring and gradually tend to stop working over a number of months and years. However, what struck me was an even more important concept that Professor Kennedy had developed in his work, namely, the ability to record from the human brain and to analyse the electrical recordings to work out what a human subject wants to say. By recording from the parts of the brain's motor cortex concerned with the muscles used for speaking, he had managed to work out (using complex signals analysis techniques) what the subject was trying to say.

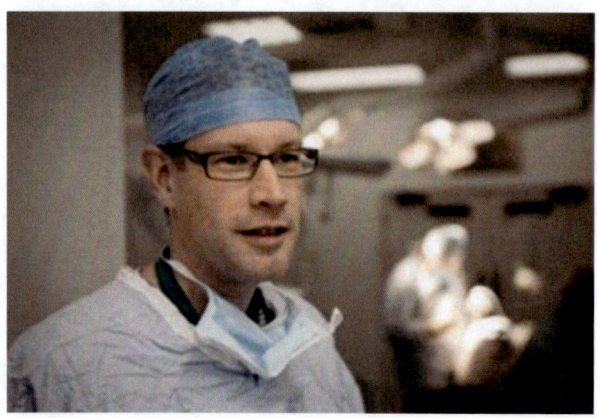

Anyone reading this book will realise that this is far more complex than it sounds (no pun intended!). Despite the fact that I am involved in neural interfaces and signals analysis, I remember being awestruck by what Professor Kennedy had achieved in such a short time. The very fact that this had already led to treatment in a patient such as Erik heralded a new era of 'bionic implants' to compensate for disabilities involving the brain that had hitherto been written off as untreatable. It was clear to me that Professor Kennedy is one of the great pioneers in this field, combining his deep knowledge of neurology, neurosurgery, neurophysiology, mathematics, engineering, and of course his innovation, ambition and blue-sky thinking.

In fact, this book has come at an important time in the evolution of the brain-machine interface. The 'Brain Gate Project' to allow tetraplegics to control robotic arms, wheelchairs and computers is well underway with important early results. In the UK, in 2019, the Royal Society has just produced a booklet called 'iHuman' which is a perspective on 'blurring the lines between mind and machine' and talks about technologies massively expanding, overtaking pharmaceuticals in their efficacy.

It calls for the UK to develop a 'Neural Interface Ecosystem' to accelerate development of these technologies, and also talks about the need to control ethical and social dilemmas such as who decides who receives these enhancing technologies. At the same time, in the US, Elon Musk is running 'Neuralink,' a start-up with an incredibly ambitious 'top down' approach to neural interfaces involving implantation of over 3000 hair-like Electrodes inserted into the brain by a robot. Clearly this is going to be an important space for development over the coming decades and will allow treatment of conditions that we have never been able to touch with medication alone.

Unlocking Erik tells the story from the human side – both in terms of Erik himself as the subject, and Dr. Kennedy as the pioneer. Those wishing to enter the domain of neural interfaces should read this book as they will learn much about how it should be done. It is a journey of quiet and slow discovery. It has taken courage and risk from all sides. From Erik's point of view, deciding to have an implant in the brain which was one of the few parts of his body that was still fully functioning. From Kennedy's point of view, starting on the project with the belief (and a very educated prediction) that it was possible, he staked his reputation and career on it. And Kennedy has gone one step further. Whilst medical literature is littered with pioneers who have tried out their own remedies on themselves (such as Giles Brindley and his implant to overcome erectile impotence which he demonstrated to a shocked audience at the Urodynamics Society conference in Las Vegas in 1983!). Even so, not many would go as far as having a craniotomy and an experimental Electrode array put onto their own brain! This took a huge amount of personal risk and faith in his work and indeed he had to travel to Belize as the US would not allow such a procedure in a healthy person for purely experimental reasons. Nevertheless, as in the other aspects of this project, the hunch paid off and important and useful data were obtained. I would predict that the field of Neural Interfaces will expand rapidly, helped by current investment such as that from Musk and others. However, for me, one of the big messages from this book is that there is plenty of space in the field for everyone, including individual pioneers with innovative ideas, enthusiasm, working from the 'bottom up' with pragmatic solutions, and courage. And there are plenty of human subjects, like Erik, with the gumption to be on the receiving end of the devices. And, just occasionally, there are those like Kennedy who blur the lines and transiently cross to the other side, bridging the gap between the pleas of the injured and the promise of new science.

Professor Alexander Green

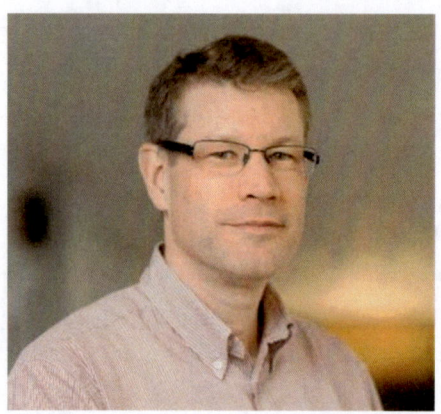

Professor Alexander Green is an academic Neurosurgeon at the University of Oxford in England. He performs Deep Brain Stimulation and other types of 'neuromodulation' for movement disorders and pain. His main research interests include the use of neural interfaces to control the 'autonomic nervous system,' including blood pressure, heart rhythm and breathing. He is currently running a trial of brainstem stimulation to control these symptoms in patients with multisystem atrophy.

Preface: Decades of Opening the Door to the Mind

When a brainstem stroke or spinal cord injury prevents the injured person from using the human body's highly evolved communication system, a core boundary has been breached: for the damage effectively severs one's thoughts from being physically emoted. And let's be clear: without our amazing progress to communicate facts, feelings, thoughts and emotions, we lack the most singular achievement of the human species.

The scientific term – "locked-in syndrome" - applies to nearly all patients in full paralysis for whatever reason. It defines the most devastating aspect of their condition: without the input of specially trained therapists or the intervention of advanced AI computer support, there is no way for them to communicate with the "outside world."

Within the great macrocosm of paralyzed victims, there are degrees of being locked-in. As you may have seen in the biographical film "The Diving Bell and the Butterfly," journalist Jean - Dominique Bauby was able to describe his life before and after suffering a massive stroke that left him with locked-in syndrome by actually creating a *memoir* from his hospital bed. He did so by blinking his left eyelid whenever the therapist pointed to the desired next letter, amid a frequency-ordered French alphabet chart. Bauby created every word, every sentence, every paragraph his book in this way. In March 1997, two days after completing his memoir, he died of pneumonia. But his book went on to become an international bestseller, and cultural touchstone throughout France. All this was possible because he could open and close his left eyelid!

You can see a variant of the locked-in condition in the life of theoretical physicist Stephen Hawking, who was stricken with ALS while still a student at University, and would suffer through his body becoming totally paralyzed over the course of several decades. But Stephen Hawking refused to accept the full mantle of being locked-in.

When he lost his ability to use his vocal cords, he and his team at Cambridge developed a computer-controlled voice-generation device, first activated by a finger-push, and then, when Hawking could no longer move his finger, activated by shifting his cheek muscle. In the ensuing years, Hawking collaborated with top experts in his field, became a leading authority on black holes, penned three international best sellers of popular science, and, when he died in 2018, was one of Great Britain's most honored scientists. Hawking lived and worked with his disease for 50 years, and maintained communication with the outside world by being able to move a tiny facial muscle.

Screenshot from Documentary, "The Father of the Cyborgs."

I'm not certain how much I was inspired by courageous individuals like Bauby and Hawking, but my own 33-year journey to understand and break through locked-in syndrome was underway at the same time they were struggling to survive and to be *heard*. From the early days during my decade-long trials with rats and monkeys, I felt certain I could fabricate a method to tap into the brain of the locked-in and give them a new option for real-time communication.

Up to this time, I had conducted solid years of research, recording with pin (or tine) type Electrodes which are stiff, insulated except for exposed tips for recording and placed beside neurons or neural processes of some kind. Our experience showed that signals would not last beyond a few hours. Improved versions such as the Utah array have lasted months or years, but then lost 85% of signals at the three year milepost, a failure for the long-term survival of the signals. But was there a better solution?

Researcher Aquayo and his colleagues in Montreal in the early 1980s showed there could be a different solution. They actually grew neurites into slivers of sciatic nerve placed in the brain. So I simply placed the slivers of sciatic nerve in tiny glass cones, placing recording wires inside and presto! An Electrode that survived the life time of the rat! My first Ah-Ah moment.

After that, monkey implants provided long-term survival of neural signals that were functional as well. My second Ah-Ah moment! After that, FDA approval for human implants (All this is described in more detail in the part 2 scientific section of the book).

Our first subject, a 59 year old woman, showed that she could control the neural signals voluntarily at our request. This was our third Ah-Ah moment! But, unfortunately, she had terminal ALS and died 76 days after implantation. Even so, she showed us the system was safe and she could control the neural signals.

Working in the Veterans Hospital in Decatur Georgia, my second locked-in research subject was the *world's first cyborg* because he could control the computer using his neural signals, thus bypassing the use of his limbs. He was able to spell his name, our names and move to targets on the computer screen. He showed that not only was the system safe, but could be very useful too.

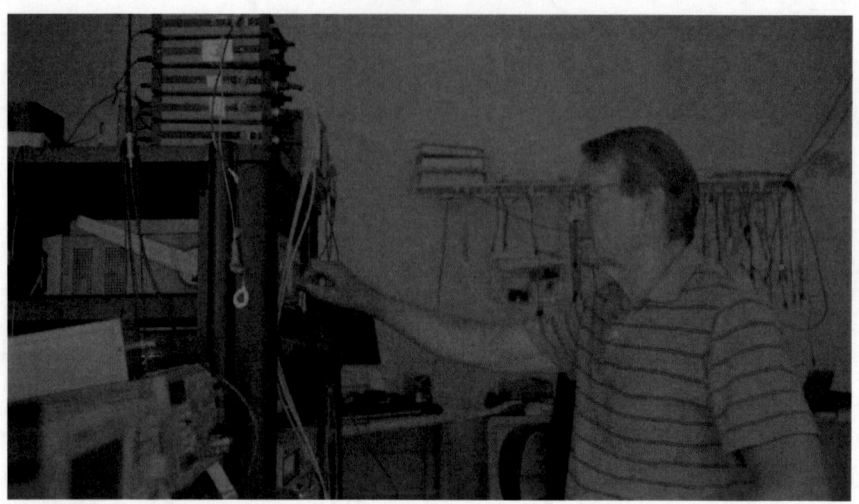

Screenshot from Documentary, "The Father of the Cyborgs."

Shortly after this, Eddie Ramsey of Duluth Georgia introduced me to his son, Erik. Erik was almost totally locked-in. He had some eye movements, up for yes and down for no. But not much else. He was in his early 20s, totally paralyzed and totally mute due to a brainstem stroke. This I felt was the ideal patient for attempting to restore speech. But little did I know what I was getting myself into!

At this point, there had been progress in this field over several decades, but not really any great leap forward. Let's go back to 1970s. A neuroscientist called Eb Fetz demonstrated that monkeys could control individual single units recorded from their brains. So I hypothesized that we could attach words to single units and Erik ought to be able to control them. As you will soon see, and in the associated video on the project website (www.neuralsignals.com), we achieved this goal.

He was able to control single units to say Dada, and another unit to say Mama. This was exciting for him and us but it also made me realize that to produce 100 useful words reliably we would need to record 100 single units and we had only achieved 40, and not all of these were useful. Also my knowledge of how the brain works led me to believe that it is *the patterns of firings* that determine speech, not just one single unit attached to one word. So we changed course and looked for the patterns of firings. We mapped the single units firing patterns onto phones, and found that about half the 39 English phones could be identified.

We then collaborated with Professor Guenter and PhD candidate John Brumberg from Boston University. They took a different approach in order to train Erik to control the cursor as it moved over the screen and produced the vowel sounds.

All this, including a video for reference, follows in part 2. The first time he succeeded in doing this we were all present and we all cheered loudly in the lab. I must admit that was not what serious scientists do, but again it was another Ah-Ah moment, so please forgive us!

Throughout a decade of working with Erik, we realized one issue was that we did not really ever know for sure when he was speaking, and when he was not speaking. So I needed a subject who could speak and then lose his or her speech over time and see if we could compare the signals when spoken out loud and when speaking silently. I was sure that nobody was going to volunteer for that. So I volunteered myself!

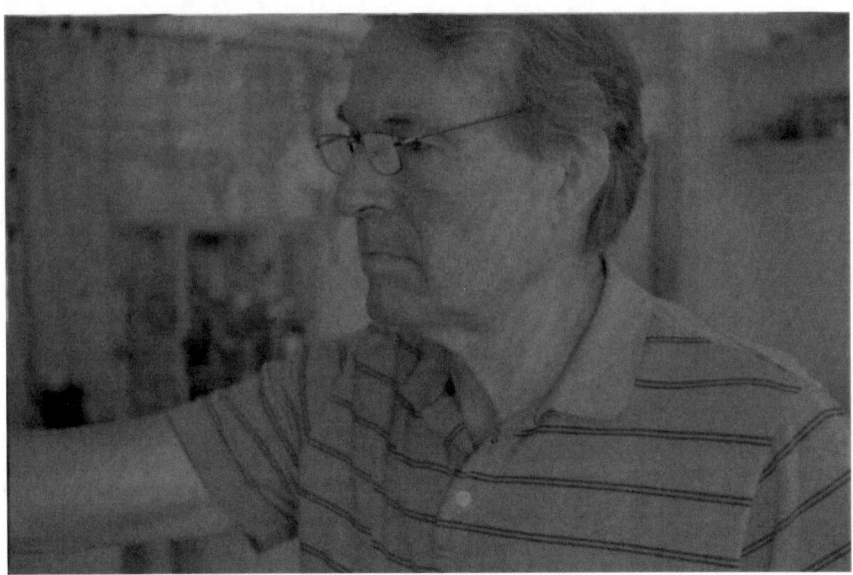

Screenshot from Documentary, "The Father of the Cyborgs."

The data that I obtained from my own brain and the use of newly discovered neural net computing paradigms allowed me to decode audible speech and silent speech. This is an important result because it means that locked-in people like Erik would be able to speak again.

What I did not anticipate was all the "lessons" and locked-in related insights I would collect over the years, and now ready to share. Nonetheless I've developed an acute appreciation of what we can call the "here and now" of the locked-in person. You will see me use the term "here and now" throughout this chronicle as my way of recognizing both the presence and the absence of the conscious interplay within our environment that we all have and rely upon *each day of our lives.*

Think about that: Our "here and now" is how we manifest being alive and aware, and being able to interact with our multi-dimensional world. We must remember that though the locked-in may very well be *alive* and *aware*, they very much *cannot* participate in the simple pleasures of living, at the very boundaries of inner and outer expression:

So …… imagine a world without all our "human" moments:
- no words of encouragement to the four-year-old child transfixed by a purple and green Hummingbird;
- no words of thanks to the friends and family assembled to let you know they are "with you";
- no whisper of love into your son or daughter's ear …
- No unseen secret shared in an intimate moment, sweetheart to sweetheart, in a language no locked-in person can use -- no matter how much their own heart aches to say it.

So think of you as them: you are unable to make a sound, render the gesture, or participate in the multilayered language of shared thought. You'd have no interaction with the moment, or, another's mind. No here and now, no transformative meaning leaping from your mind, through emotions, to the senses, and beyond… Because there is no "beyond" if there is no way "out into the world."

So "unlocking Erik" is, in a way, also a look at my own journey into the mind, in order for there to be a journey out of the mind. You will see me and the brave individuals who are willing to have the Neurotrophic Electrode implanted in their brain involved in an act of "**defiance**"; their act of saying "this locked-in syndrome *does not define me,*" and it is not a *life sentence* to a world of lost interactions and confined feelings. But naturally, the earlier test subjects would not have the degree of potential change that subjects today may expect!

Unlocking Erik is my way of showing that locked-in syndrome *is simply not part of the life we are designed to experience.* We need to change our thinking about it to a more transformative science and creative art, even to a transformative love that can redefine how we sometimes become hurt and broken and try to put ourselves back together.

As essayist Parker J. Palmer has cautioned us about misunderstanding *human wholeness:* "**wholeness** is the goal, but wholeness does not mean *perfection.* It means embracing brokenness as an integral part of life."[1]

And dare we say it, *A life that love and belief can transform.*

---

[1] Parker J. Palmer Essay on Wholeness. *On Being* broadcast. July 8, 2015.

ACKNOWLEDGMENTS

First, I thank Bruce Mitchell for placing the idea for this book in my head. Second, I want to thank my wife Joyce Houser for tolerating my questions and reading the text. Third, I want to thank all the excellent neuroscientists, engineers and neurosurgeons who made this effort possible, including the late Dr. Roy Bakay, Andre Joel Cervantes, Princewill Ehirim, Brandon King, Joe Wright, Jessie Bartels, Kim Adams, John Goldthwaite, Melody Moore Jackson, Todd Kirby, Steve Sharpe, Dinal Andreasen, Thomas Wichmann, Frank Guenther, Jonathan Brumberg, Mark Clements, Brian Mathews, Celeste Ramos and Meel Velliste. And finally, this book could not have seen the light of day if it were not for Brian Shaw, ghostwriter extraordinaire.

The research described in this book was funded by the National Institutes of Health and by the author.

Income derived from sales of this book will be devoted to research for unlocking the locked-in. A small percentage will go to Erik's family.

Part 1: Erik's Journey

Chapter 1

BREAKING THE SOUND BARRIER

"For millions of years, mankind lived just like animals. Then something happened which unleashed the power of the imagination. We learned to talk and learned to listen. *Speech* has allowed the communication of ideas, enabling human beings to work together. **Mankind's** greatest achievements have come about by talking and his greatest failures by not talking...."

--- Stephen Hawking
for British Telecom, 1993.

"My diving Bell becomes less oppressive, and my mind takes flight like a butterfly."

--- Jean-Dominique Bauby
The Diving Bell and the Butterfly

After nearly 25 years of working with paralyzed victims who have lost their ability to communicate, it's now clear to me that perhaps our most valuable human trait is the one that appears whenever someone decides *not to give up!* A decision to fight back against unforeseen tragedy, standing against devastating misfortune, or standing up to a relentless enemy. I've seen firsthand terribly injured individuals face overwhelming adversity and say simply: "*I will not give up.*"

This also tracks with the fact that often our most vaunted cultural heroes are not great warriors or top athletes, but the heroes whose compromised bodies still can't hold back the ignoble spirits and determined hearts of these individuals.

24 – Karat Courage

In fact, it would be hard to think of anyone with more of a claim to our popular imagination than the late theoretical physicist, Stephen Hawking, and the French journalist, Jean-Dominique Bauby. Both Hawking and Bauby had debilitating, profound paralysis thrust upon them without warning and yet both managed to not only deal with the loss of locomotion and unassisted communication, but dramatically transcended these physical plights and heroically broke through their "sound barriers" and produced books that were international best sellers. The world at large seemed to pause a moment, taking in how two men with locked-in syndrome both refused to accept this death knell on regular forms of speech and writing, using one of the smallest muscles of their bodies to reach the attention of medical therapists and so begin with tiny building blocks of language -- a single letter or word -- to produce a book.

Hawking's *A Brief History of Time* sold an astounding 25 million copies, translated into 40 languages. While **Bauby**'s *The Diving Bell and the Butterfly* -- a memoir of his life before and after becoming locked-in, was written from his hospital bed: he blinked his left eyelid whenever his speech therapist pointed to the letter he wanted her to type next as she traveled her finger along a frequency-ordered chart of the French alphabet: *E S A R I N T U L O M D*.

His "Butterfly" appeared about a year later in France, and was anticipated by a few small reviews in the French press. However, neither Bauby nor his publisher was prepared for the reaction of the public: the first printing of 25,000 copies sold out in a single day! By the end of the first week of publication, "The Diving Bell and the **Butterfly**" had sold 150,000 hardback copies. And of course, the posthumous film of his book won awards all over the world.

Certainly physical and intellectual achievements such as these – from amid a cold and dark condition – got my attention from the perspective of my university research. From where does the almost unbelievable level of resilience and determination stem for one to accomplish these personal triumphs? How does one summons the faith and strength needed to transcend what had long been thought of as "insurmountable" odds?

I wanted to know and understand the psychological and spiritual mechanisms at play when a locked-in individual ignores their cruelly severe limitations. And I wanted to do this at the same time I was focusing my scientific career on understanding the mechanisms in the brain that I could tap into, attempting to "reawaken" the individual communication system that was so suddenly shut down. One of the first things I needed to prove was that, within these individuals in their desperate, locked-in state, their ability to communicate *was just lying dormant, but not destroyed.*

When Bauby asked, rhetorically, "Does it take the harsh light of disaster to show a person's true nature?"[2]

I thought, well maybe: it depends upon whether we can cheer for ourselves to never give up, or, if that is not precisely in our nature, then, the cheers of others must surely be weighed and counted.

For Bauby, who received hundreds of letters during the months he labored on his memoir, it was both. "[Sometimes] the letters I received simply relate the small events that punctuate the passage of time: roses picked at sunset … Or the laziness of a rainy Sunday. [It is] these small slices of life that move me more deeply then [official pronouncements]. I hoard all these like treasure. One day I hope to fasten them end-to-end in a half-mile streamer, to float on the wind like a banner raised to the glory of friendship."[1]

Just as France had so opened its heart to Jean-Dominique Bauby, it felt like half the world had embraced the travails of Stephen Hawking. And this, despite how, early on, the prognosis by his medical team in England offered

---

[2] Jean-Dominique Bauby (2008), "The Diving Bell and the Butterfly," Vintage International, Vintage Books, Random House, New York.

very little encouragement. At age 21, Stephen was given just two years to live unless he committed to using a ventilator.

Diagnosed with Lou Gehrig's disease, a degenerative motor neuron condition that attacks the spinal cord and central nervous system, he would ultimately face ensuing paralysis, eventually shutting down his entire body. Yet, while the onslaught of an incurable disease would stop most in their tracks, Hawking redoubled his efforts in theoretical physics, and relied on a large network of contacts, researchers and assistants to support his determination to continue teaching. For the next 15 years he held weekly classes and conducted new research in quantum physics, and then, at age 37, became the Lucasian Professor of Mathematics, one of the most prestigious positions at Cambridge University. So prestigious, that in the 17th century, that same title was entrusted to Sir Isaac Newton!

But when Hawking contracted pneumonia in 1985, he could not breathe on his own, and rather than be tied to a life-support machine 24 – 7, his medical team performed the tracheotomy allowing breathing through an opening in his throat. Unfortunately, the procedure left him unable to speak. Even when he could only whisper words to a personal assistant who had allowed him to carry on with his classes, this was different. He told reporter Ed Bradley that "For a time after my operation, I was devastated. I felt that if I could not get my voice back it would not be worth carrying on."[3] But once again, that 'special something' that these heroic individuals draw upon in times of darkness was ignited, and Hawking turned to voice synthesis technology and challenged his computer colleagues to build a computer that would give voice back to a beautiful mind, however slowly it operated.

While I did not have a hand in helping Hawking or Bauby, I did embark on a decade long effort to restore the speech of a locked-in teenager named Erik Ramsey. And now it is time to unlock his story.

Thanksgiving week, 1999, 16-year-old Erik Ramsey lay motionless in the intensive care unit of a Lawrenceville, Georgia hospital; while he'd survived a devastating car crash, he had lost his ability to communicate. A

---

[3] "The 60 Minutes Interview with Stephen Hawking." 2003. CBS Television Network.

brain stem stroke caused a debilitating condition, disabling all control of his muscles, shutting down his speech and any use of his limbs.

Erik had survived the accident in one sense, yet his family could see no evidence of the personable, creative, humorous teen he had been. They could not break through the barrier of silence stifling his speech, nor detect anything "alive" about his lifeless form as he just lay there --- locked-inside. In fact, the technical term for this medical condition is actually called "locked-in syndrome."

Being "locked-in" like Erik is horrible, but it is not a death sentence. Erik's mom Sandra Ramsey, holding his hand by his bed, knew that Erik was *not dead inside*. Perhaps this is why Erik's family intuitively clung to the hope of some cutting-edge medical intervention, even *before* they had spoken to the hospital neurologists and physical therapists on his odds of ever making some semblance of recovery.

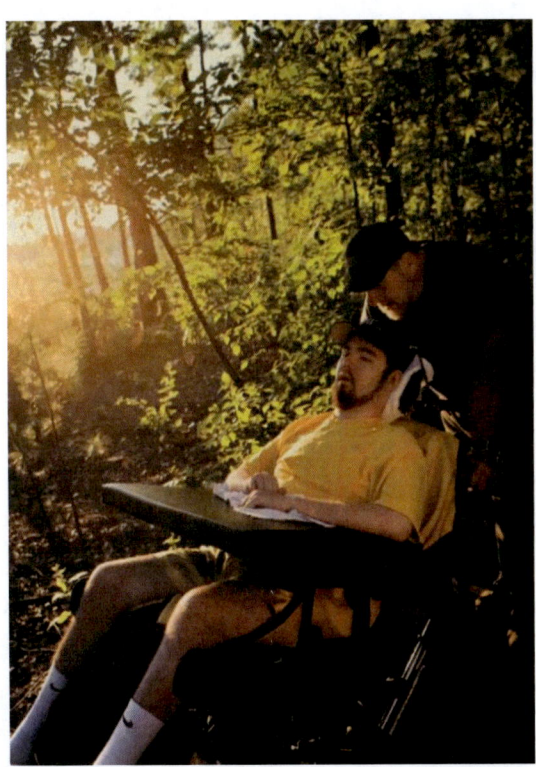

For locked-in patients, their condition can be seen as a "ventilator dependent disease", but not a fatal one if a ventilator machine is used continuously. Even so, though they are kept breathing --- *kept alive* --- by the machine, they are still a person who is *present*. They may not move or speak, but there is a person who can think clearly and also feels emotions. Not having the physical use of their body does not wipe out their humanity! Yet, we sometimes wonder: can they think clearly and deeply?

Yes! Just think of the late Stephen Hawking, renowned astrophysicist and cosmologist, *locked-in for 50 years*! But that did not keep him from mastering theoretical science and proving a thousand naysayers wrong as he went on to fully collaborate with other scientists, like physicist Sir Roger Penrose on gravitational singularity theorems that they would later turn into award-winning research. Or, his producing eight best-selling popular science books, or, his participating in a dozen films and documentaries about his life and work.

Through a combination of bad-ass willpower and an almost super-human ability to look on the positive side of any equation, Hawking's life is a rare but seminal example of mind over body, heart over hurt, and positive over negative energy.

For this was *not* a case of a famous expert in his field being cut down later in life: Stephen Hawking learned of his dire straits at age 21, still in university and during the early successes of a brilliant mind. But he processed the startling medical diagnoses with his own version of *Pascal's Wager*: he decided he might as well intend to excel in his chosen field anyway, not in light of early, widely held high expectations, but rather, because now he had to let those go and endeavor to go *beyond expectations*. He told the New York Times "my expectations were reduced to zero when I was 21. Everything since then has been a bonus".

Hawking *accepted* the horrible realities he faced, which allowed him to look beyond them, and into a universe of unfathomable possibilities.... He seemed to know and believe his future would hold even stronger, more positive realities. *It was the simple grace of hope and the extraordinary belief in one's self.*

BREAKTHROUGH

Fortunately for Erik --- and his family --- over the ensuing weeks between Thanksgiving and Christmas, an unexpected but *crucial* grace note appeared concerning his locked-in predicament. One afternoon, his hospital-based speech therapist noticed Erik had control of his upward eye-movement. Amid the vast mechanical abilities of the human body, raising the eye vertically is the smallest, most quiet, physical action that can take place. Yet this one, tiny "micro gesture" could allow him to answer simple "yes" or "no" questions, *in real time*. Real-time communication would offer the building blocks of *real time conversation*.

Erik Used to Write Books as a Child

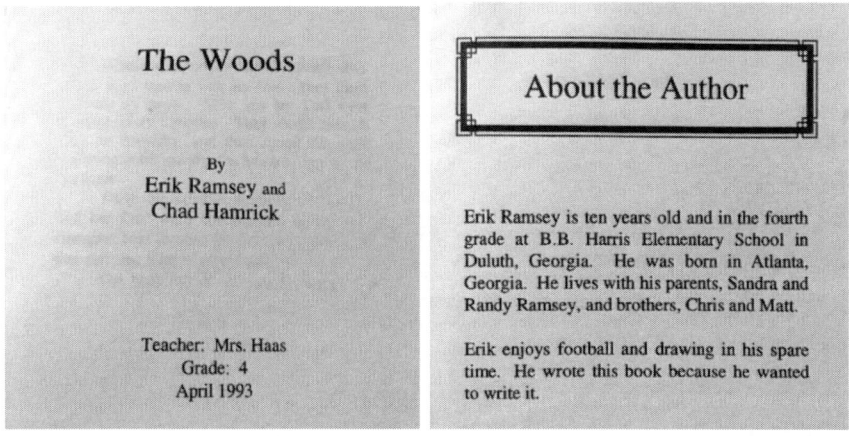

The full impact of this tiny discovery may not have been apparent that afternoon, but the fact that Erik would be able to make at least one "articulatory gesture" would be a game changer! It offered a breakthrough into that barrier of silence, if ever so slightly!

After several years of clinical therapy and home care, when Erik's father, Eddie Ramsey, contacted me at my Neural Signals office in Duluth, Georgia, less than a 10-minute ride from their home, he did so armed with that new bit of hope. I'm a neurologist and neuroscientist specializing in brain computer interfaces (BCI), and Eddie knew this "opening" into Erik's locked-in condition and relatively stable condition would get my attention.

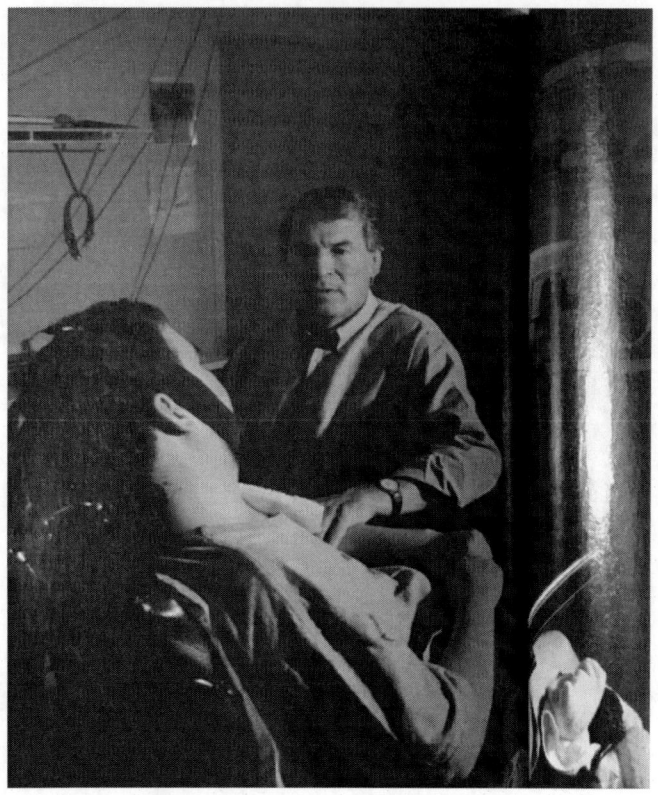

Since 1986, I've been developing methods to apply BCI hardware directly to the brains of locked-in patients, utilizing a device I invented known as the *Neurotrophic Electrode*.

Harnessing the neural dynamics of patients' brain activity, my team has been developing a system for speech generation that uses neural signals that are amplified and then sent to nearby equipment which runs computer algorithms capable of identifying the right sound phone or word that the patient is only silently selecting.

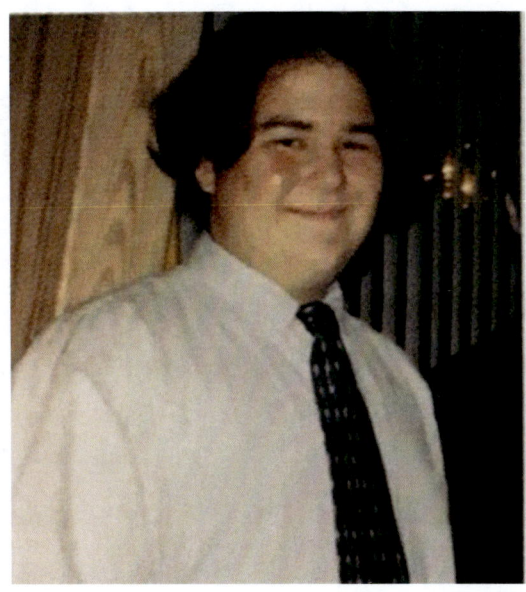

Erik, one year before he became locked-in.

No one was saying it out loud, but conceivably, if we successfully synched Erik's attempts to make sounds (that is, his actual "trying" to speak in his head), with the BCI support equipment, he might become the first patient in the world to have a thought pattern successfully interpreted by software and rendered into speech in real time through voice synthetization.

In a few days, Erik and I would embark on a never-before-realized journey through space and time, trial and error, and fits and starts. One that would try the very limits of patience, endurance and determination of us both!

Though the basic concept can be stated simply: the patient tries to say words while the brain machine interface translates that attempt into speech, the needed man-hours of research, testing and experimentation to accomplish this goal remained a vexing unknown. It would be another decade before new discoveries in artificial intelligence and deep learning might solve some of the problems of identifying the brain's speech locus --- even if the individual is *not* speaking out loud.

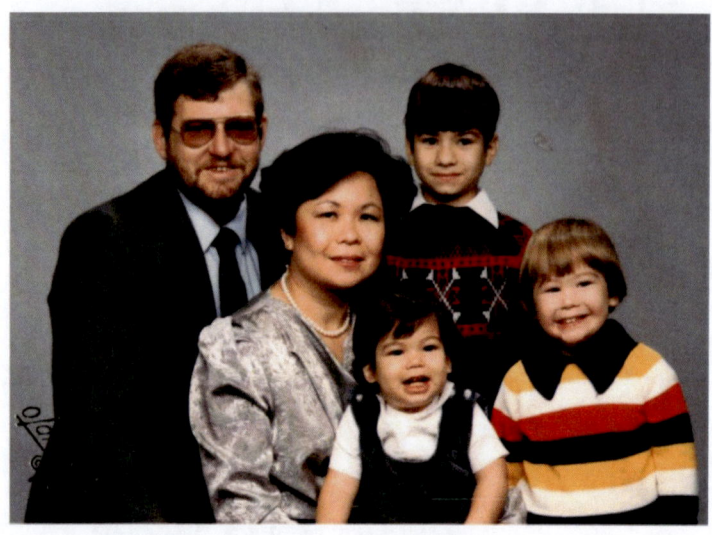

The Ramsey family: Erik is on the right, Mathew is in his mother Sandra's arm, with Eddie and his older brother Chris.

HEARING A PIN DROP

Visiting the vast and mysterious *meadows of the mind* is a journey I have been making for nearly 50 years now, basically since medical school so many decades ago. Mapping areas of the brain in order to allow the study and repair of various brain functions has been my scientific pursuit for many decades. It can be conducted with highly specialized neural imaging equipment, that, when supported by additional data processing, maps behavior or intent onto specific brain regions. Or, it can be attempted during an actual brain surgery operation, by interacting with an awake and aware patient who gives feedback to a neurosurgeon's stimulation of selected regions of the exposed brain (This is possible because there are no *pain* nerves extant in the human brain's neuropil).

Originally undertaken to identify areas of the brain that control movement of the body, in order to help investigate the possibility of repairing damaged areas of the body, more recently identifying the speech areas of the brain has become a dedicated field of research. As neuroscientists agree on naming and cataloguing discrete regions of the brain, the prospect of sharing such research across scientific disciplines is becoming a reality. One team of investigators has, for example, delineated the area for controlling the articulators, and has pinpointed the exact location on the brain map where neural patterns form into words by driving and controlling an array of articulators, -- your tongue, jaw, cheeks and vocal tract. In this area, combinations of scores of tiny neurons fired this way or that, forming the individual phones that are combined to make words, and words into sentences.

It may help to keep that level of detail in mind, as we learned Erik would have to start his new speech process by learning to envision the *individual sounds* that brain functions carefully assemble to form a *single word*. So the formation of speech begins with the formation of discrete sounds, but done in milliseconds, if not nanoseconds. For Erik, we would be attempting to restore the functionality of speech at a smaller and more elemental level than even a baby uses to learn to talk!

For us to be successful on this journey, it will be incumbent on Erik to access his strongest personality traits --- especially, his intellect, creativity and sense of humor. It is said that intelligence is the ability to adapt to change, and I cannot think of a more challenging acid test of this concept than the determined skills and inner fortitude needed for Erik to will his participation in this attempt. For him to break through this barrier of silence that currently locks him away from friends and family, and in effect pulls an iron curtain around his "here and now:" his ability to really live "in the moment."

Chapter 2

SOME SUPERHEROES ONLY FLY INSIDE

"For men must never feel a cause is hopeless – [a soldier] must never feel an enemy cannot be beaten!"

--- Stan Lee

In the first popular superhero comic books, Superman and Batman battled the 'forces of evil', relying on their super-human strength or state-of-the-art crime-fighting gear and gadgets. Ironically, it was also their superpowers that soon made their storylines a bit too predictable. It was not until Stan Lee established his more troubled, "anti-hero"' storylines a few decades later at Marvel comics, that mainstream comics experienced a renaissance: for Lee understood that the most compelling and relatable superheroes *are the ones that are most human.*

I had been thinking a lot about human and superhuman capabilities the week I would meet Erik Ramsey and his family, compelled to weigh the pros and cons of Erik's locked-in syndrome in relation to my ongoing research aimed at enabling paralyzed persons to transcend their paralysis. (At least to the point of being able to communicate through a next-level brain computer interface).

It was clear as new crystal how intensely Erik needed, and wanted, to break through his shroud of silence: he teetered on a relatively slender timeline of hope for a successful brain implant procedure. Already profoundly immobile and mute, with Erik's condition we would have no baseline of speech and limb failure to track and plot, as you might have had with many ALS subjects like, say, Stephen Hawking when he was not yet fully paralyzed and with no complicating cognitive dysfunction. To work with the intricacies of human speech at such a basic and critical level, and to do so having to utilize only partially understood cognitive functions that allow and support that speech, I would need to use and continue to refine, state-of-the-art "decoding" software and equipment that, fortunately, had just been developed.

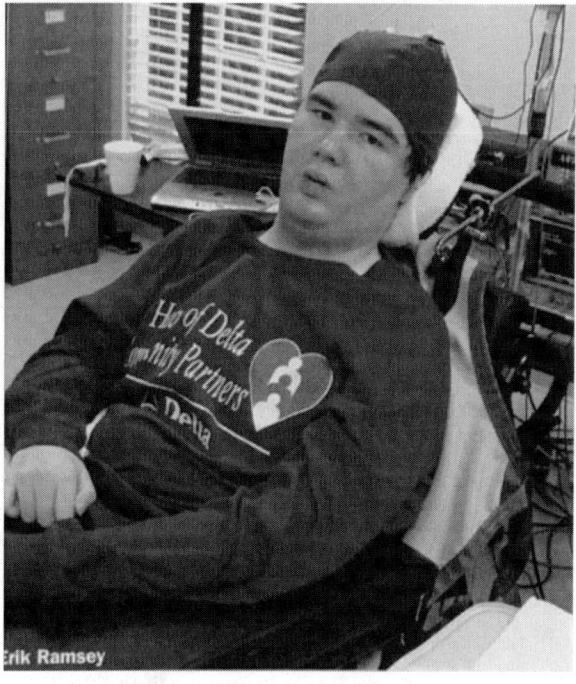

We would need to identify and capture Erik's "trying to talk" brain signals into a consistent neural data stream, and then use our surgically implanted Neurotrophic Electrode to direct the signals to amplifiers secured under Erik's scalp and capable of sending the signal through the scalp to the decoding equipment nearby.

In a kind of closed-loop feedback we would be starting with Erik's thought to say a word, and end by either having a display screen show the word or the sound of a word, or, have a synthesized voice generator approximate the sound Erik was thinking about, into the room in real time.

Fortunately, I knew from my research over the last decade that the precise placement of brain implants would be crucial for the recording equipment to succeed with the level of accuracy that could allow speech recognition. This is not some random exchange of electrical information from brain activity, but rather an attempt to communicate *knowledge*; the actual words, or the actual phones used to form words Erik intended to "say." For example, think about how many different words there are in the English language that are only three letters long and end in "at." The phone or micro sound of 'b' makes "bat," and "H" makes "hat" and "c" makes "cat." And where would we be if Erik suddenly chose to quote some William Shakespeare (we would need specialized algorithms loaded with *Elizabethan phones and phrases*!)

> "That time of year thou mayst in me behold,
> when yellow leaves, or none, or a few, do hang,
> upon those bows which shake against the cold,
> Bare ruined choirs, where late the sweet birds sang."
> --- W. S. Sonnet 73

Deciding whether or not to take Erik's case, I faced an almost overwhelming range of extremes: beyond his "ruined choir" of complete loss of speech and muscle response, were his still troubling crash injuries - compromised lung and blood pressure function - going to halt our experiment or delicate brain assessment procedure without warning. A *single cough* could disrupt and skew the recordings during neural signals decoding, for example. Other troubling and very real "unknowns" concerned both his stamina and his frame of mind. There could be years of demanding, painstaking lab sessions needed to permit him to master the support equipment interactions and mental agility necessary to regain any semblance of routine communication. Would Erik be up for that?

Obviously, the makeup and performance of his "support team" was no small consideration. They might literally make or break Erik's limited chance for success. Anyone who has sat at the bedside of a friend in hospital understands how relentless and demanding the smallest human needs can be. For an immobile person even a sip of water or change of bedclothes can be a daunting, deceptively difficult, multi-person happening. Erik was going to need a true team of *"superheroes"* surrounding his every day existence, helping defy the hurdles and roadblocks already imperiling the way ahead. Could they do that? Was it even possible?

GAMES OF CHANCE?

So, I would be rolling the dice on Erik with only my data and experience to say: "Go ahead! Roll them!" But rolling them *felt right.*
So I did.
Fortunately for me and Erik, both he and his dad were *fighters!* Both of them valued the confidence one needs to excel at sports, cram for an exam, or be willing to go against the grain of rules and protocols if that's what it took to be heard, or stand up for your rights. And though it might first appear counterintuitive, one thing Erik had going for him was almost 20 years of loving football and wrestling, cheeseburgers and fries, teenage girls and Japanese amines, and the action-centric memes of *Power Rangers*, *Dragon Ball*, and sci-fi films. As I began to get to know Erik and Eddie, I was learning how devastated they both felt at his *loss of self*, and how determined they would become to fight back and reclaim it.

In a strange way, I began to see Erik's near-total loss of humanity with reverse logic: it somehow made him *more human*, because he was so painfully aware of what he had lost! I began to see that every time Erik's dad fought the hospital staff or insurance companies to get him more therapy, or make him more comfortable, it was a "father and son tag team", their way of saying these human plans and failures were not the norm: "normal" was everything that Erik had unwillingly given up, held at bay for the moment by cruel circumstance, but still clear in Erik's and Eddie's memory and heart.

So then, could I help Erik *not* accept his current 24/7 reminders of a life lost, and instead, offer the hope and challenge of the even more important things we could fight to bring back that could change his present reality? For the tragically injured like Erik, the bias of *presentism* is the most severe: The shock of what has happened can crowd out any positive thinking about moving forward and actually disable our capacity for hope and forgiveness.

Erik needed nothing less than a reason to go on living, and the belief in our eventual success. Could I give him that? Could the math, science, the Electrodes and algorithms of my lab develop a *new normal*, and just maybe, rekindle that pilot-light inside each of our hearts? I believed both Erik and Eddie were up to the challenge, and that was good enough for me.

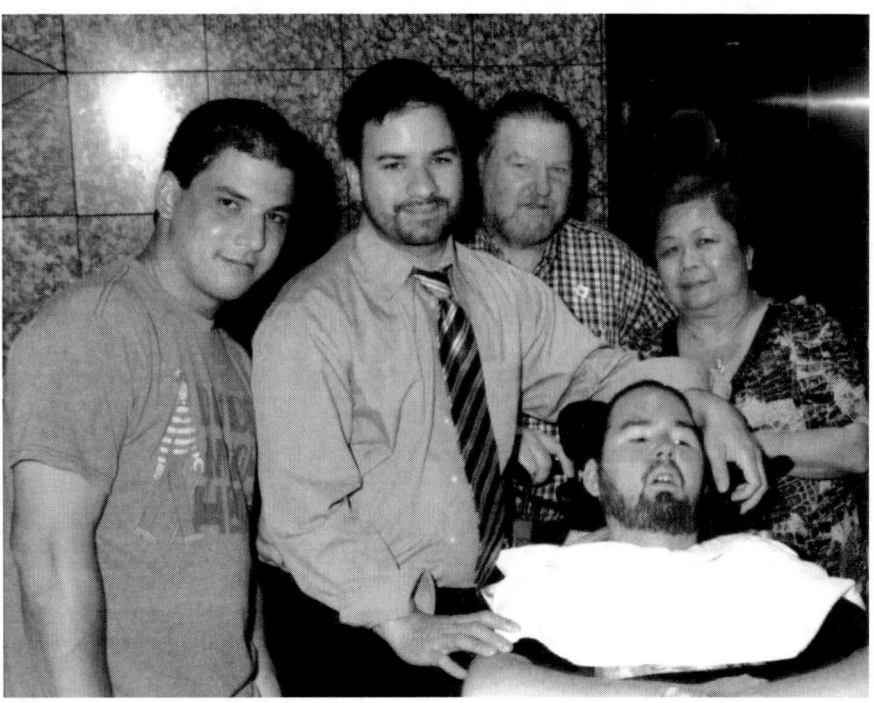

Erik's brothers, Chris and Mathew with his Dad Eddie and Mom Sandra.

Chapter 3

CODING AND DECODING ERIK'S INNER DIALOGUE

"… The passion of being was in thinking, and that comes from that two–in–one dialogue in one's head. That … [is] … the beginning of moral life … If you can't have that inner dialogue, then you can't speak and act with others either."

-------- Lyndsay Stonebridge, on
Philosopher Hannah Arendt,
as told by Kristin Lin, onbeing.org

After preliminary talks with his family, I first met Erik Ramsey at his home in Duluth, Georgia. I remember being struck by how silent and motionless he was. Our first communication: he gave me an eyelid lift for "yes." I noticed his left eye did not look straight at me, and his right barely moved in its socket. His "no" was simply eye down and eyelid closed. I explained the project to Erik in as simple terms as I could: the goal was to use a computer screen and possibly a synthetic voice generator to display Erik's words and thoughts in as close to real time as possible. We would be implanting an Electrode on a specific activity area of his brain, and then fitting his skull with amplifiers covered by his scalp that could boost and send his neural signals to nearby equipment that would decode the signals and render them into the basic elements of speech. Erik listened and gave me his "eyelid up" *yes!*

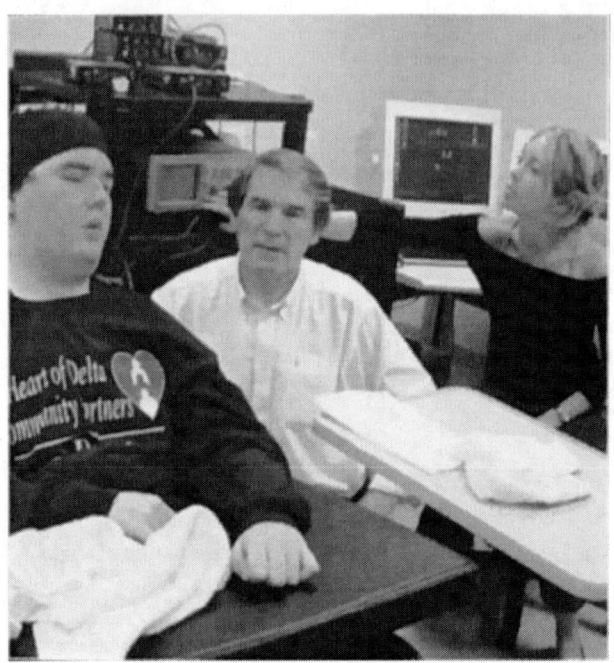

Erik, myself and assistant, Jessie.

When I got back to my lab that afternoon, I sat down and wondered: was Erik the right person for this research? Did I really know if he could understand enough about what would be required of him? When he had the stroke at the hospital before going home, what happened to the rest of his brain? While I could run tests to learn more, we still had background constraints I was more than a little concerned with: Does Erik have seizures? Even the onset of a partial seizure could interrupt and be deleterious to the nascent interpretations we would be making from our first data. Equally important, I had to ask how disappointed would he be if this was a total blowup and nothing worked? Indeed: I knew my Electrodes were sturdy and dependable and would work. But what about the tiny electronics? I knew they should work and could be changed-out if needed. But I also had to admit that the Electrodes could not easily be changed out surgically. That could be a deal breaker.

These were all very lucid second- thoughts and timely ones. Apart from Erik's onboard technology we had carefully tested our decoding equipment that would separate out his continuous data stream into single units, convert them into *phones* (the building blocks of language), or whole words, and then use these to playback his efforts.

Earlier that day, I had ended my talk with Erik trying my best to emphasize the difference between what our *goals* were, and what I could actually promise him:

- I could promise him the completion of the Electrode surgery;
- I could promise him weeks of recovery time, possibly with troubling side effects, such as lung infection and blood clots;
- I also could promise him the need for concerted efforts to learn and interact with the computers and the decoding system.

And that would be a process lasting years!

It was well to keep in mind, also, that this was something of a "second chance" for Erik and Eddie, on their quest to return his facility for speech in real time. Erik had stopped using the phone / word chart so carefully designed and set up by his dad in his early recovery after the accident. It's potential for accuracy was countermanded by the profound fatigue it would bring to bear on Erik. So my *Neurotrophic Electrode* was both a second chance, and possibly, a last chance for Erik's speech.

Our goal was nothing short of turning the most destructive moments of Erik's life into a *path of transformation*. With anything less in mind, I don't think I could have moved forward, and I don't think Erik would have been interested.

Setting aside whether or not we ever "deserve" the mishaps and injustices that befall us, whenever an *inciting incident* succeeds in totally disrupting the balance of our lives, we are also given an opportunity to transcend previous boundaries and raise our game. I wanted that for Erik and his family. Fortunately, despite my concerns, Erik's brain MRI showed normal hemispheric structure and his EEG (electroencephalogram) had normal background brain activity with no suggestions of seizures. I decided to schedule his surgery, and after careful monitoring during recovery, we established his first sessions in my Neural Signals research station. Erik had begun a journey to reclaim his speech!

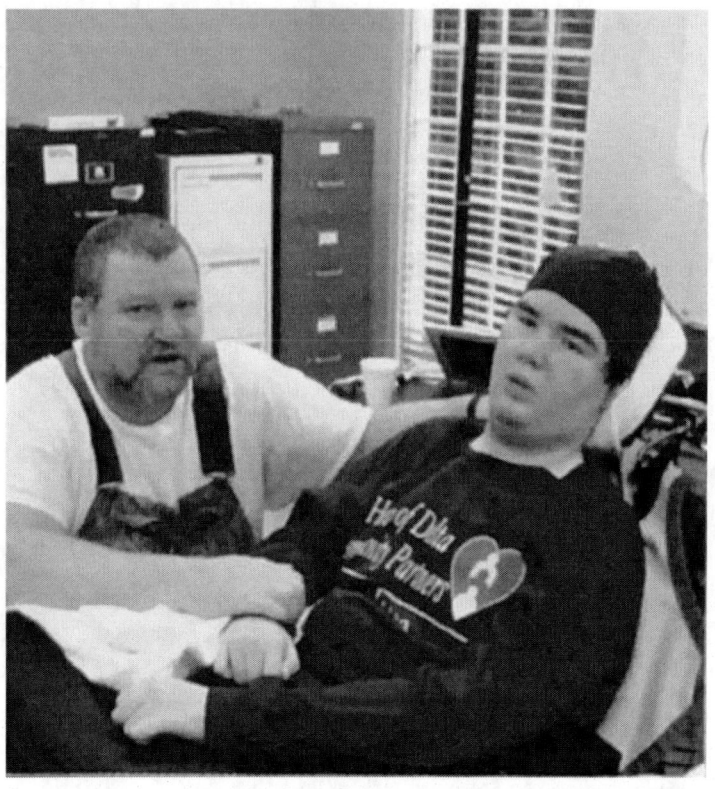

Entry to the lab was easy. From out of the van it was flat all the way through the main floor and into the 20 x 30-foot recording room. The equipment was basic but very serviceable. Erik was wheeled into the room and backed up to the bank of controls. We mounted the coils on his head to power up both the implantable amplifiers and FM transmitters. During the recording session, a power coil and FM receiving coil were adhered securely to his scalp using C2 water soluble EEG paste.

The support equipment behind his wheelchair included FM receivers, tuned to a frequency that ranged between 35 and 55 MHz, and external amplifiers that could send Erik's processed signals to speakers or unprocessed signals to the recording equipment. A DDS digital tape recorder archived our data stream, and customized software separated the signals into two streams, both filtered to help standardize the data and minimize the effects of noise artifacts that could skew the data analysis.

Our working sessions in the lab were set up partly to support research by Jon Bromberg of Boston University. This allowed the single unit data to be routed to another computer, so that an LDA software paradigm could drive the mouse cursor over the screen controlled by Erik's neural signals. The computer screen display was projected onto the wall facing Erik, allowing him to both *see* the cursor move and *hear* the vowel sounds he was generating. This step alone was a significant move forward in BCI research, and I hope Erik knew how significant his participation was even at this early stage.

Erik's surgery for the Neurotrophic Electrode and support electronics took place in September 2004, and went smoothly, with several weeks for healing and recovery. Our team included Dr. Princewill Ehirim, neurosurgeon, of Gwinnett Medical Center, Lawrenceville, Georgia, Stephen Seibert, Edward Joe Wright, Jessie Bartels and myself, at Neural Signals.

This was the first operation anywhere in the world for the purpose of implanting that exact configuration of glass cone and gold-wire filaments directly under the surface of the pre-motor speech cortex, the area that controls how our jaw, mouth and tongue interact to form words as we speak. While scientists had probed parts of the brain in motor function location experiments, ours was the first team to believe a single implant system could provide full or partial speech. From the perspective of pure science, we were -- truly -- on the first step of the thousand mile journey. For both Erik and myself, I realized the most formidable challenge would be to not let the inevitable setbacks that lay in wait for us dull our spirit, or derail our determination.

Beyond the Call of Duty?

Despite my years of preparation for this, and having a leading-edge team on-hand for Erik's operation, as the first recording sessions were underway in early 2005, it soon became apparent we had a component failure in one of the tiny electronics that supported the implantable Electrode. There was no silver lining tucked inside this, our first major setback. Simply put, we would have to take Erik back to the operating room and replace the tiny support electronics. While I had total confidence in my Electrode design and fabrication -- their base components of glass and Teflon insulated gold wires were sturdy, and their construction was dependable -- my only fear was that in changing out the electronics, the Electrodes might become damaged: the only way to remove the electronic connectors attached to the two Electrodes is to drill away the cement -- a very delicate procedure.

Chapter 4

BELIEVING IN THE MAGIC, COUNTING ON THE SCIENCE

"Set your life on Fire,
And seek those who fan your flames ... "

Rumi

SPEED AND PATIENCE

Scene

Inside the dome of a rollerblade sports arena ... as a vocal crowd cheers on individual skaters:

ERIK is in the lead, the steady strokes of his legs pushing him forward, like pistons in a sports car engine. He swings out in a wide arc, then *SWOOSHES* back by the bleachers, where about 50 of his high school classmates snap pictures or raise their hands and arms in a frenzied wave of "high-fives". He is like a *blur*. As he comes around again, he *leans in*, lowering his head and making his head, neck and shoulder muscles like the tip of an arrow, in flight along the arena.

On every wall in the background, giant murals display the cartoon characters from the *Dragon Ball* Japanese amine TV series, as overhead, huge speakers hang from the rafters, blasting out the main theme song from *Dragon Ball* by the pop star Hiriki. Erik lowers his crouch even more, pumping his legs even faster now, *syncing* with the beat of the theme music, leaning ever forward, almost at the tipping point ...

Then, on the next pass, he swings back out to the far wall, then pulls close in again, as he approaches the bleachers ===

=== I can see a distant gleam in Erik's right eye as the orderlies push his hospital bed into the O.R., and I wonder *"where does he go"* when he is not focusing on the questions I have put to him in our research sessions, or, when pushing away the pain he must feel when we interact with him, trying to add a moment of touch to his immobile body?? *Where indeed does he go?*

Erik's mom, Sandra, had said once that Erik admitted to having a special place he went when he closed his eyes and stopped trying to connect with those outside his mind, but also said he'd never tried to spell out where the place was. But I had an idea, based on his years as an athlete, love for rollerblading and fondness for the unlikely heroes that make up Japanese amine. It would be quite a spectacle, with Erik in the middle ... In my mind, I could just see a rollerblade dome in the distance ...

We had just rolled past Erik's parents heading to that "repair operation" to change out the faulty electronics that short-circuited our neural signals-to-Electrode speech sessions. And yes, my heart probably hit some extra beats as my colleague Dr. Princewill Ehirim drilled the hardened glue off of Erik's Electrode connector.

But the electronics change out went smoothly, and after two weeks of rest and recovery, our new sessions mapping Erik's neural signals and their nanosecond journey to the sounding of phones got underway in earnest. It was to be a decade-long odyssey, trying the patience and endurance of Erik, his family, and myself. And as that song says: *"I wish I didn't know now, what I didn't know then!"*

Working with tragically injured, locked-in individuals, trying to simply rekindle their most basic abilities to have communication and human interaction, does not allow you to make room for "happy ever after" scenarios. Or even, someday seeing them reacquiring any type of normalcy in their personal, everyday lives.

Clearly, Erik and his support teams were facing many years of both trying to maintain the fragile health he had, while at the same time, trying for some modest, weekly incremental progress. As we experimented with the neural signal firing - speech activation points in his brain, we endeavored to establish a lab-specific communication process that would at some point allow him to be less locked-in. Within this landscape of trying to avoid setbacks as we sought to maximize his unknown potential to improve, there are actually two "tracks" of routine challenges:

One, times of physical set-back, with Erik's family taking him to hospital; two, more fortunate times where months of sessions in my lab slowly began to unlock some of the secrets surrounding his brain -computer interface possibilities and limitations. He "see-sawed" from progress to unforeseen burdens …

Those first years after Erik's car crash evidenced how far Eddie and Sandra Ramsey would go to fight to retain some semblance of Erik's pre-crash life: Erik loved wrestling and once a week the Ramsey's invited some of his closest friends over for pizza and "Wrestling Night". Other routines that offered Erik a bit of a "to do" list included his brothers watching "Power Rangers" and "Dragon Ball Z" with him.

When Eddie discovered his son's eyesight was weakening and glasses were a chore to deal with, he brought home a giant screen TV, and Erik became something of a *cinephile*, watching film favorites like *JURASSIC PARK* several times a day. But by the second and third years, post-Electrode implant operation, Erik's health declined, and these neighborhood "activities" gave way to a new pattern of clinic and hospital visits.

THE STATUS OF NO STATUS QUO

The trips to the hospital became longer and more frequent. Another major challenge to the Ramsey's was that it became apparent that many hospital staff had only minimal training in the care of quadriplegic's who are also mute. On days when they had to check in to the ER, family members had to ensure that at least one of them was on hand to oversee his complex medication and supplement schedule, teaching nurses how to utilize the vibrating therapy vest that kept Erik's lungs from collecting excessive fluid levels, not to mention a half-dozen range-of-motion exercises and special throat-suctioning equipment. Falling off schedule with either his meds or his liquid nutrients could cause dangerous blockages and blood pressure changes that could turn the quiet start of the day into an afternoon of extra nurses on hand, with careful monitoring of his vital signs, monitor alerts and warnings.

For our research with Erik at Neural Signals, a constant challenge from year one to year 10 was *to understand the variability of his neural signaling*, and to develop consistent parameters wherein we could measure and accurately interpret Erik's neural speech activity. Of course I did not achieve the research at Neural Signals by myself! I had a great team of problem-solvers working alongside me.

Computer programmer Edward Joe Wright came on board in 2005, helping to decode Erik's selected phones and words by using a software paradigm called Support Vector Machine. This neural net algorithm allowed the decoding of words and sounds off-line. Helpful though it was, the calculation density of its instruction grade were not fast enough to use online.

But in 2009, Prof. Frank Guenther and Jon Brumberg came to Neural Signals labs from Boston University to adapt an online algorithm called Linear Discriminant Analysis (LDA). Though not the performance numbers I was hoping for, its faster processing allowed Erik to move from vowel to vowel over the computer screen. As he used the system, he could see the cursor move and hear the vowels produced by the various cursor positions on the screen. So we saw real-time progress in working with Erik to bring him back into his speech process (Years later, I would learn to appreciate this step as one of our hard-won goals).

So for example, Erik could make and move from vowel sound 'aaah' to vowel sound 'eeeh'. Although we were still not at the speed of functional speech, this was significantly faster than using "see and point" letter chart or including an interpreter question and response step. Week-to-week, year to year, *the question was always how much speech can we decode in real time?* I had to balance our need for speed with the *almost painful reality of Erik's physical interactions*. He was thinking some of the smallest gestural steps of human communication, and he was also "out there," continuing on his quest to replace silence with meaningful sounds.

Chapter 5

UNEXPECTED DELAYS AND EUREKA MOMENTS

"A failure is not always a mistake. It may simply be the best you can do under the circumstances. The real mistake is to *stop trying*!"

---- B. F Skinner

I took on Erik's case at the halfway point in my career. Nothing in my early research on the Neurotrophic Electrode, or even the subsequent research on Brain-Computer interfaces with partially paralyzed subjects, prepared me for the challenges, frustrations and expectation-crashing realities that morphed into our weekly lab routines during our decade-long journey to help Erik Ramsey regain his patterns of speech.

This went beyond research "**conundrums**", like why must it always be "two steps forward, one step **back**," with progress in the research lab? If you can't accept that level of necessary patience, then **don't** be a scientist! But this was different: this was having to accept a new normal of endless and unexpected setbacks. It reminded me of a piece on the "First Flight" by a heavier-than-air aircraft, the Wright brothers "Wright Flyer" flight on December 17, 1903, in Kitty Hawk, North Carolina. The reporters said what was remarkable was not that they got 20 feet off the ground in a sustained flight, but that they got 20 feet off the ground in a sustained flight after failing to do that 200 times before. According to biographer David McCullough, Wilbur and Orville Wright understood the importance of how we frame our experience: they would crash their plane, and then they would say: that was *great!* I know what went wrong! Every crash became one more mystery solved. I began to wonder what exactly should our measuring stick for "success" actually be in locked-in syndrome research? Would we look back someday at Erik's newly regained "conversations" or would we look back someday at the *number of times Erik thought about talking?*

Wherever you look at the icons of achievements in World History, you see testaments to "stick-to-it ness" and perseverance. Einstein once said he wasn't smarter than fellow scientists, but that he would chase after a problem longer than they would. Decades if necessary. We read interviews with individuals who are tops in their field, and often the most profound point is all about *attitude*: Bruce Lee once said: "do not pray for an easy life. Pray for the strength to endure a difficult one." I wondered what Lee would think of Erik's quest -- ready to climb a mountain to say a word! Maybe we did need a new scale to judge our progress by, after all.

At the heart of my journey with Erik and his family was our ongoing mandate: *to see how much speech we can decode in real time using our brain computer interface,* providing a locked-in individual with a real reason to think about communicating again.

On the plus side, our "proof of concept" was proving itself in the early going: the Neural Brain Signal – to - Electrode – to - amplifier – to - transmitter – to - software processing model not only works, but promised opportunity for real time, lab-time, incremental improvements as we move forward with software enhancements and more nimble and sensitive lab equipment. On the other side of the ledger, it was equally true -- and equally confounding -- that an almost unfathomable number of real-life interruptions and unforeseen hurdles sprung across our path. Granted, events like the sudden collapse of electronic components in the B – C interface are possibilities research teams must "factor in" to their expected goals. Parts fail, and expectations held while undergoing brand-new scientific procedures must stay at arms-length at best.

Also anticipated -- with a cup of coffee and a couple of aspirin -- was the likelihood of misleading electronic artifacts from false readings: we'd seen the induction coils slip off target on Erik's scalp causing those voluntary signals to be distorted or completely lost.

But on the flip side of these *anticipations* we had to dig out the needed *determination* to respond in kind: if the hurdle seemed a little high, maybe we needed a lighter track shoe. Early days, those amplifier coils were held in place by a stretch-cap over Erik's scalp. But our much simpler new approach - to secure the coils with a dab of EEG paste -- did the trick, and held them in place far better. One hurdle passed! Even so, our next session could just as easily hold a new pitfall.

One recurring delay stemmed from the fact that roughly half of our sessions with Erik would hit during a time when Eddie had no choice but to step in and feed Erik through his stomach tube. Eddie had a feel for the best feeding timetable for Erik's system, and there was even a link between an infusion of nutrients and Erik's energy level and concentration. But the feeding tube could also disrupt the readings we were getting, causing us to start over. And the ensuing steps to then suction his mouth and throat added more interruptions.

LEVELS OF MAGNITUDE

Sometimes the recurrent challenges to our sessions were at a whole other level of magnitude: they arose from classic, unanswered questions of hard science that were seemingly hardwired into our research model.

The most unexpected upset was when we realized that the *firing rates* of single units were not consistent. We had noticed in a previous project several years earlier that when we were preparing to set up the equipment, his single units fired actively. But minutes later when we got down to work they were quiet. This happened repeatedly and I thought we lost the units to some component failure, but then they became active again while further working with the subject.

So with Erik, we noticed the same thing: we realized that we were on a "sea of waves,"; sometimes the waves were high and the single units were active; sometimes there were low and there was no unit activity. This was very upsetting to our having any firm sense that we were getting good readings, I realized that we need to do an in-lab test study.

We had Erik sit quietly in his wheelchair as I turned off all the lights, encouraging him to deeply relax -- or even go to sleep. The units in the B – C interface quieted down, especially in channel 1. Everyone was quiet and I watched and waited.

But then the Eureka! Moment for me appeared when his dad unexpectedly entered the room. As Erik recognized him, the neural firings increased dramatically. We soon did some control test to show that it was not just the movement in the room, lights or change in background music. We showed that this powerful response was purely *emotional*.

This was a breakthrough moment: in other words, we learned our emotions can determine what wave we ride on in this turbulent sea of neural activity. Just like the windward lift, or push on a sailboat in open water, with high emotions neural activity is higher, and with low acquired emotions we settled in the bottom of the wave, with corresponding low activity. These results have been published and are described in part 2 of this book. It seemed a bit counterintuitive, but I learned that we can assume we have reached the core level where problems originate, only to find that *there are deeper levels still.*

INNER TRUTHS?

Each time we had a lab session, I was poised and ready for our team to establish just the right B – C interface specs and unlock Erik's "voice" and so break the invisible chains that held him back. I would look at Erik, motionless in his wheelchair, patiently waiting for us to reset the "PAUSE" button and restart his life.

If only I could say -- with Michelangelo, that "I saw the angel in the marble, and carved until I set him free."

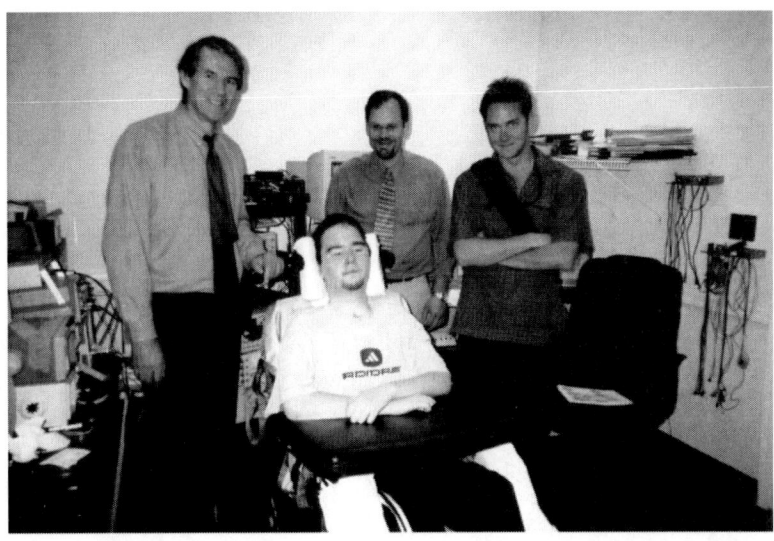

Erik, myself (left), Roger Miller (NIDHC, NIH) and Joe Wright (programmer).

Chapter 6

THE PLACE WHERE "I" EXISTS

"[Be still] ... the trees ahead and bushes beside you are not lost. Wherever you are, is called 'Here' and you must treat it as ... powerful ... must ask permission to know it and be known."

--- David Wagoner
"Lost"

When I came from Ireland to North America, I was leaving the green hills of the medical school in Dublin, for the giant pine trees surrounding the University of Western Ontario in London, Ontario, Canada. In fact, I'd be taking my residency on a campus sequestered by shade trees as old as the city itself. Though newly married and transplanted to this new country my "sense of place" hadn't changed that much.

At the medical College in Dublin I was keenly interested in the function and still – hidden mysteries of the human brain, and was the "go-to" guy when fellow students needed to understand how the brain worked or the blueprint of its capabilities. No surprise: I have always pondered ways man could maximize the brain's potential through bio – technical enhancements --- the place and a process for conscious knowledge and consciousness might converge and force - multiply the brain's capabilities. That's why as a young physician I returned to school to earn a PhD in neuroscience.

THE FAR HORIZONS

This is a vast field, from the imaginings of "super humans" proposed by decades of science fiction writers, to today's proponents of Artificial Intelligence (AI) dominance --- like Ray Kurzweil and Marvin Minsky. My own research eventually focused on one aspect of this field: could a B – C interface jumpstart the possibility for those with debilitating paralysis, *intercede* and unlock the mind's landscape of expression? Developing such a Brain - Computer interface always struck me as an almost humble, attainable, near-term goal, particularly in a near term future where experts envision all knowing supercomputers like the HAL 9000 in Arthur C. Clark's and Stanley Kubrick's *2001*, and now with Kurzweil adjusting - forward his prediction for *technological singularity* to 2029, where the limitations of our biological bodies will no longer be a factor. They will seamlessly morph into the architecture of a next - level brain machine.

In fact, Kurzweil believes that the reason so many think of his Singularity event as something in the far future is that such an exponential technological achievement is "counter - intuitive to the way our brains perceive the world, since our brains were biologically inherited from humans living in a world that was *linear and local*," and as a consequence, he claims it has encouraged great skepticism in his future projections.

So I asked: can we tap into the act of thinking and knowing that is always being expressed in the pathways of the brains of paralyzed individuals? If the answer is "yes", then we can intercept the signals and decode them with software support. But in order to get to that "here", we first had to get "there", and for a decade or more I took the time - worn steps of testing my theories, in the lab, with peer-reviewed animal trials.

I landed an academic post at Georgia Tech, a research university in Metro Atlanta, where I did my initial experiments with Long Evans rats, accessing the motor cortex brain waves. It was also at Tech that I developed the first glass-tipped Neurotrophic Electrode, which allowed me to implant the device into the cortex of Erik's brain. Here, the solution of growth factor cocktails inside the tip promoted the growth of Erik's brain tissue neurites *into* the inner chamber of the glass tip implant, thus ensuring a safe and stable nesting of the device. This "growth factor" step solved the problem of dislodged implants that other researchers had and still do experience.

Then, to refine the design of our implant components I experimented with a special breed of monkey at the Yerkes Primate Center near Emory University. This animal testing culminated in FDA-approval to finally implant the Neurotrophic Electrode into the subjects where extreme paralysis had precluded any other means of real - time communication. This "go ahead" with human trials allowed me and my colleague, neurosurgeon Roy Bakay at Emory Hospital, to focus on profoundly locked-in candidates.

NEW OPTIONS AND OLD FEARS

A Vietnam Vet at the VA hospital in Decatur, Georgia, Johnny Ray had suffered a debilitating brain stem stroke, losing the use of his four limbs and muscle responses over 99% of his body. But he retained eye-movement and a slight muscle movement around his face and neck, and this small opening allowed JR to be an "ideal" candidate for our Electrode implant trials.

Over the course of months, and after allowing for the nesting and stabilization of his Electrode implant, we worked for several days a week to teach him to control the computer cursor by first *thinking* of moving his arms. (We had implanted his arm area.) This eventually led to Johnny being capable of "action thoughts", in effect, utilizing his brain signals to activate the next cursor move by just thinking of the cursor and not thinking of his arm! When the media learned of this breakthrough, Johnny Ray's story became headline news, and both Dr. Bakay and myself were interviewed by major newspapers as well as morning news magazine programs. This milestone went way beyond "proof of concept" and signified real progress within the field of BCI technologies. But JR's pain threshold was soon into an area that was not manageable with mid-level painkillers. He was often actually too sedated for communication sessions to continue.

Another year passed, the JR media headlines echoed a while and then died away ... And then a 16-year-old boy named Erik came very close to being another highway fatality on the nightly news: when I learned of Erik's case, and the Ramseys decided to go forward with the operation, I had no way of knowing that between JR and ER, 15 years of my professional career would be swept along the wave of neural signals, decoding the intentional firing of the brain's will to communicate. We looked for signs of non-static neural sparks in the search to *decode thoughts* – – an approach not unlike how SETI's search for Extraterrestrial Intelligence scans the heavens for radio waves with profiles that don't match the ongoing noise and interference always present in atmospheric reception.

Looking back now, I wonder at all that time "waiting" for baseline "quiet" times in sessions when no extracranial disturbances would muddy the waters of our signal analyses. In JR's case, it was a challenge to find intervals where his level of pain had ebbed enough for him to be hooked up to our equipment. In Erik's case, it was the number of technical adjustments necessary to ensure his sessions yielded usable data: we had to progress from using single-Electrode points to drive his sending short words like "Ma" and "Da", which he mastered quite well, to the much more complex approach of "studying *patterns* of single unit firings". We would need hundreds of the single unit "events" in Erik attempting to talk if we were to ever allow him to fill in the elegant yet simple mosaics of human speech. It was all about harnessing those signals!

So, here I was with Erik. Our sessions reaching intermittently across a decade. And though it was never a formal or scientific concept tied to our working sessions, there seemed to emerge an additional context to our work, an additional way of *thinking* about what else might be achievable.

The deeper my work gets into understanding and orchestrating the control of BCI and support devices, it seems the closer I come to understand the "here and now" of a locked-in subject trying their best to be human in their suddenly inhuman reality.

The "interpersonal" space, say, between two people, that language can bridge and energize, becomes a gaping *chasm* for locked-in individuals – – a "here" without any solid ground, or "common ground" between them. Like a no-man's land, even one devoid of the continuous chaos the rest of us feel when we are *not* talking.

I realized that, too often, to be "here" for the paralyzed and mute is to really be nowhere, at least without the countervailing caring and intention to reach out across the chasm by another caring individual. And if there is no here to be in, then where is one's *home* as well?

We can get a sense of just how much a locked-in individual loses when they lose language by taking a moment thinking about how crucial it is that we be able to access the power of language and infuse words with a bit of who we are as a person.

Today, in Ireland, there is a poet and theologian named Padraig O'Tuama who has spent more than a decade among those who deal with the aftermath of the "troubles" in Northern Ireland, in troubled places trying to help both Catholics and Protestants heal and learn to speak a new language of compassion and understanding. Something he discussed recently with ON BEING's Krista Tippett. From the controversy surrounding so-called justified killings at the borders, to evolving concerns on community standings on gay marriage and self-rule, O'Tuama has spent thousands of hours meeting and conducting dialogues intended to show the power of language at work, creating new *heres* and *nows* that can bridge the chasm of fear and ignorance. Mindful of the problems we can experience when symbolic language and political "**trigger words**" are used without careful consideration, O'Tuama explains how shared language needs "**courtesy**" and "**generosity**" to guide it, and can curate "**inclusion**" into its potential for meanings between the lines -- when those lines actually may define what here and now can become. He calls this being *attentive to the implications of language*, and believes that with enough care and wisdom we can give language an air of sacrament.

If we have no "here" to share with another, as befalls many locked-in individuals, there is no way to be with one another – – life's most cherished and taken-for-granted blessing. For Padraig O'Tuama, being able to *belong* is what "**creates** and **undoes us**". Even with a profoundly locked-in soul like Erik, we must learn to go beyond even the precious gift of speech, and ask and learn: *"How are we to be with one another?"*

Each morning we begin anew:

"I wake.
You wake.
She wakes.
He wakes.
They wake.
We wake….
[And it is up to us] To take this troubled beauty forward". [4]

As best we can.

---

[4] Padraig O'Tuama, "On Being" with Krista Tippett.

Chapter 7

DEEP PRESENCE: UNDERSTANDING THE HERE AND NOW

"When we are *connected*, each of us is able to be more *fully alive*. Poetry finds and gives voice to these connections. But as we keep trying to inhabit the possibilities we carry within us, we're inevitably stopped by the fires of experience that burn down the temples we have built ... "

--Mark Nepo
"The Necessary Arts"

In the last chapter, we began to get a sense of just how much a locked-in individual loses when they lose language. Accessing the *powers of language* and conveying thoughts and emotions with it, forms a huge part of our humanity: exchanging feelings and imparting solutions to everyday problems nurtures our *emotional intelligence.*

Beyond this, in our concept of "Here and Now" we are adding-in the interplay of real time interaction with our environment. When our consciousness is engaged, our awareness kicks into overdrive, and all the senses connect with the world around us, and the "being" inside us.

A Meaningful 'Here and Now'

When a medical event causes an individual to become locked-in, the aftermath is a wide wake of broken connections, work-around routines and a greatly diminished quality of life. With special research participants like Erik Ramsey, with whom I was exposed to more than a decade of his friends' and family's coping mechanisms and constant support, one sees both the profound physical loss, as well as the widely important, tiny moments of *transcending* his affliction: His obvious pleasure and responsiveness to hearing a guitar chord from the rock band Slipknot is one I will never forget. Erik became "animated," but of course, the locked-in can't become animated!

If one respectfully sets aside Erik's pain, physical loss, and voiceless existence, what is left are the dozens of 'openings' that arise, moment-to-moment when we can *respond differently* and creatively to sharing communication and the moment with him.

Here is a silent one I observed in a family video Eddie Ramsey showed me when some of Erik's friends were over for pizza and football:

They pulled Erik to the center of the rec room where he had a perfect angle to look up at the large flat screen TV. Friends filled the chairs and sofas nearby. The big college game came on, and the university cheerleaders had their moment on national TV: as the camera zoomed in on the lead cheerleader, Erik's brother pressed his arm, smiled and gave him a big "thumbs up."

Using spontaneous social gestures he was *vocalizing the moment* for Erik, and with him. That *interaction* served to enhance the experience for his locked-in brother, no matter how simple or short-lived!

It may have felt counter-intuitive at first, but over time I realized that the more I saw what Erik couldn't do, the more I understood who the real Erik was. He was made of things just as genuine as writing a poem, or singing along with his favorite band, they just were not as obvious -- you had to look a little harder to see them:

You can see determination in the set of a brow or chin;

You can feel sorrow in between the return of a gaze and the delayed blink of an eye;

You can sense anticipation in the shorter pause, before the locked-in subject thinks about a special-50-yard line seats at a playoff Falcons game;

You can know the disappointment deep inside when the locked-in individual loses his ability to focus, and the energy to participate melts away, like the sudden fall of a cherry blossom.

More and more, I began to see these glimmers of Erik, however fleeting, like flashes of silver light on the heather, in the gloaming of the ever-setting sunset that was his life.

After all, these moments made up the "essence" of Erik, the pieces of soul he had left; they became the fight song for his spirit, and the lyrics to a lost love song.

THE INFINITESIMAL TRUTH

I have seen locked-in patients give up, and I have seen locked-in patients refuse to stop trying as they focus every fiber of their being on trying to move a computer cursor one letter space with their thought. In both cases, part of this "seeing" is in my mind, along with theirs, and in both cases their individual "signature" pervaded that moment, however small it might be.

In Hindu philosophy, the cosmos is replete with gods and demons who like to argue the fine points of life and death. In one instance, "Death tells a disciple about the soul: 'Concealed in the heart of all beings is the Atman, the Spirit of the Self,' he says. 'Smaller than the smallest atom, [yet] greater than the vast spaces.' This Atman, which resides in everything, is part of the essence of the universe, and is immortal." [5] If we think of all the unsaid thoughts of a locked-in, or try and sense all the unexpressed feelings, we realize there is a whole universe waiting to be experienced. And whether

---

[5] Seife, Charles. © 2000 "Zero: the biography of a dangerous idea." Penguin Books, New York, NY, pp. 65-66.

they break through the locked-in sound barrier with just a few words like Erik, or by creating a silent memoir like Jean-Dominique Bauby, they are giving us a glimpse of another world, a dimension watered by angel tears, and warmed by smiles that never quite manage to rise to the surface of their lips. A here and now that only manages to bloom when both the locked-in individual, and the person in their presence, protect the dignity of the moment by having faith in that "unreadable compass," the human heart.[6]

When essayist Parker Palmer says you must "unravel the story you tell yourself, in order to discover the story you're [actually] in," [7] he hints at the pervasiveness that telling a story or listening to a story has in the unfolding of our lives.

REINVENTING YOUR STORY

> "Listening [is] a commitment to exploring and building connections with others based on our shared humanity, even when that kind of connections *seems impossible.*"
> Andrew Forsthoefel
> "You are either listening or you're not"

Of all the maladies and illnesses that may befall us as human beings, the most disturbing must be the day-to-night transformation of a healthy individual into a locked-in one. The shock, for example, of seeing a lively, athletic youth like Erik Ramsey morphed into a near- lifeless, immobile body in a hospital bed in the space of just a few hours is dumbfounding --- almost *unbelievable* to the family of the injured.

A Navy veteran I know once shared these lines of verse; he had found them pinned to the bulletin board in the lobby of a VA Hospital:

> "My shining hour is over;
> whatever I was, I am no longer.

---

[6] Nepo, Mark. *The Way Under the Way,* "Breaking Surface."
[7] Parker Palmer, blog essay, "On Being."

And though you choose to marvel me,
no impressions will I leave."
Anonymous

It goes without saying that many veterans arrive in that lobby with a tragic loss of limbs, or with body parts destroyed by enemy mines and IED's (improvised explosive devices).

Whether we are talking about veterans of war, or tragic accident victims, we are talking about individuals whose lives have been so altered by events beyond their control that they must reinvent their self-image, redefine their life story, and create an entirely new way of seeing themselves in their world.

BROKEN SYMBOLS

Understanding the "deep presence" that this new self-image must embody, and how deeply it affects the injured subject, is the beginning point of how we must all learn to connect *with what is left of once whole human beings:* individuals with wounds that are such an affrontery to human life and dignity that it will take the highest awareness of everyone around them to rebalance the scales, and rekindle the situational awareness. We cannot accept, or, be part of accepting, an end to the life story due to loss of speech and mobility.

While it may at first seem counterintuitive, when they lose connection to the world around them, they can also lose their belief in self. This has to do with our facility for creative expression and the power of human intuition. Having that expression forestalled, or having that inner story generator stilled, feels like a death of the spirit. It is about losing one's symbolic storyline; how one's journey in life is interwoven with the cultural experiences one values and participates in. How events become part of the personal story of memory.

ARCHAEOLOGY OF THE SPIRIT

This is not unlike the concerns of modern-day archaeologists who are trying to cope with the loss of the oral tradition among many of the younger generations of indigenous peoples. If the young won't take up learning the details of the council fire, then the accomplishments of entire generations could be lost. No shared narrative, no storyline to carry forward the continuity of the culture. And, could we not say, no way to break through to locked-in individuals, no way for locked-in individuals to carry forward their story.

In writing about the power of knowing and sharing the stories, emerging author Carolina Hinojosa-Cisneros points out:

> "It is an honor to carry the story on your back and we hope that our children will grab hold of those backpacks, fill them with new stories, and continue to carry the old ones. This is how people survive."[8] She even believes that once such cultural journeying ceases, "We can become lost at the end of sentences ... Our history not honored."[7]

We consider this as we are considering the profound loss of language and story for the locked-in. We do honor one another with the gift of language: sharing a thought is another way of saying "I value your opinion ... or, what do you think of this ... or, how would you handle that...?

When we share a conversation in real time it is just shorthand for the larger effort of connecting the moments of a culture. Before the world-changing technology of writing and books, and the more recent media of film and television, the oral tradition was how we cemented together the actions of individuals, as well as our thoughts and reflections about those actions.[7]

The tradition became a more formalized part of the social structure as ministers spoke from their pulpits and orators held forth at town hall meetings. Traditional narratives are also reinvigorated when local gatherings

---

[8] Hinojosa-Cisneros, Carolina. "We survive by telling stories," blog. May 14, 2019. CisnerosCafe.org.

re-enacted historical events, celebrated national holidays, and special organizations like the Boy and Girl Scouts embraced the lore and legacy of their forbearers.

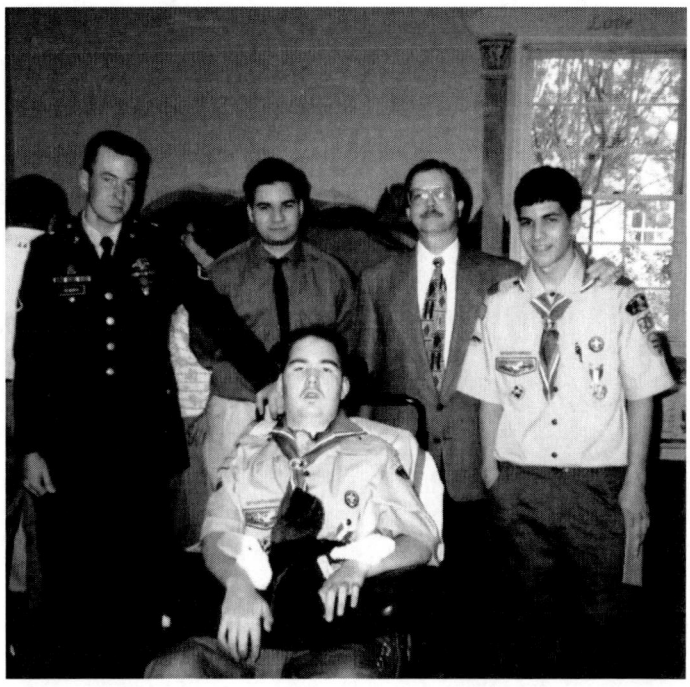

Even so, today we are in danger of losing all the rich textures of local traditions in the face of forced globalization and one-world thinking. The Here and Now of the locked-in must be capable of sustaining their individual story and affording a "deep presence" to connecting with - what is for them - an ever more elusive world.

MODERN IN NAME ONLY?

What we casually call 'Modern Medicine' today is only just scratching the surface of providing locked-in subjects with the physical, psychic, and auditory support they need to maintain their mental health and to believe they "have a future."

By adapting new tech advances specifically to the needs of individuals who have lost their ability to communicate in real time, we would be harnessing the dynamics of Virtual Reality platforms, inter-cranial music and audio, as well as hyper-sensational modalities that could very well enhance the Here and Now of the locked-in in transformational ways and with transcendent results.

In the same way that severely locked-in individuals must reinvent their personal stories, we must accept the challenge of redefining the Here and Now for locked-in subjects by expanding their options for meaningful, *now* experiences. Let us accept Buckminster Fuller's challenge to recognize the unique contribution each of us can make and even in the most difficult of circumstances:

> "… And never forget, no matter how overwhelming life challenges and problems seem to be, that one person can make a difference in the world. In fact, it is always because of one person that all the changes that matter in the world come about. So be that one **person**."

Chapter 8

THE UNCHARTED WATERS OF RESEARCH: *'HERE THERE BE DRAGONS'!*

"It is ironic but true: the one reality Science cannot reduce [or understand] is the only reality we will ever know. This is why we need art. By expressing our actual experiences, the artist reminds us that our science is incomplete, that no map of matter will ever explain the immateriality of our consciousness."

--- Jonah Liehrer
Proust was a Neuroscientist

The dark blue waters of the Caribbean rolled by Belize City beach, and from the small hill of the villa where I watched, I could almost hear the waves beckoning me to tan and tide. The yellow food carts of the food vendors on St. Thomas Street were piled high with bananas and Sunnyside egg nachos, and I could hear the loudspeakers on the neon-colored tour buses down the road.

Unfortunately, however, I might as well have been sitting beneath a dusty service station awning in Nowhere, Texas: Because I was convalescing in a guest house following a 10-hour brain surgery and found myself suddenly "locked-in:" my ability to speak and write disappeared *48 hours* after my operation.

And I wasn't dreaming ..... so, how did this happen?

After spending exactly 30 years ensuring the performance of my Neurotrophic Electrodes and their ability to safely capture the sound that the brain is sending out on its speech pathways; and after detailed compatibility tests on 42 rats, and implanting eight monkeys and five human subjects, you might think we acquired enough baseline data to verify our locked-in test subjects were being accurately tracked, allowing us to distinguish among wanting to talk, but being unable, thinking a word, and, vocalizing the word that our system processes and "speaks" through voice synethization. But in 15 years, we'd not been able to map out real speech patterns that we could then use later, as a baseline for when the same subject might lose the use of the nerves and vocal cords due to paralysis. We needed to be able to compare the brain's electrical fields when making a string of words, to a word stream generated by *thinking alone*, as amplified and processed by our Electrode-to-transceiver system.

To do this, we needed to implant a person who could still speak, and then have them "speak" both audibly and silently so we could study how the two kinds of signals were formed and used in our brain's speech processing. But finding the right partially-paralyzed subjects, who would then decline into a completely locked-in condition was proving nearly impossible, and at about the same time, the FDA stepped in and made it completely impossible: they withdrew permission for me to implant the Neurotrophic Electrodes because we could not show that the *trophic growth factors* that I used to grow neurites inside the glass tip had been proved safe to use in human trials. When I pointed to the years of animal and human tests, all conducted with no harm to the subjects, they persisted, requesting to know the formula used in the trophic growth factors.

A request I could not comply with, due to the proprietary nature of those special ingredients for the company that made them. I was going to have to send in the only pitcher who was left on the bench, and hope he could paint the outside corners of the plate like Greg Maddux, throwing his best split-finger fastball. I was going to have to pitch the game myself! And due to the FDA ruling, I'd have to do it in Belize.

I was certainly taking things to the next level by becoming the next Electrode implant subject, and a number of colleagues were aghast at my acceptance of so many elective risk factors, but, to continue our sports analogy above, *you don't win crucial games by playing it safe.* The immediate needs of neuroscientific research rarely allow for the perfect timing of crucial events: Yes! I had a wellspring of experience in working with locked-in individuals, but there were still many limitations to the knowledge about them that I had acquired. But by having my own operation, I should be able to connect a lot of dots, and fill-in areas about decoding the signals that had thus far eluded us.

"A FULL COUNT"

Dr. Atul Gawande practices general and endocrine surgery at Brigham and Women's Hospital in Boston, and is also a professor of surgery at Harvard Medical School. He also writes very lucidly on the challenges of being a good doctor in today's high-stakes medical culture. He recently discussed his book, *BEING MORTAL: MEDICINE AND WHAT MATTERS IN THE END* with ON BEING'S Krista Tippett and said this about facing crucial decisions: "… That you don't have all the knowledge, that your abilities are imperfect, that the information is incomplete, and yet, there are times when acting is the better choice than not to act. And then you live with consequences and learn from them. You take ownership and responsibility, and move on."[9]

After choosing to act, I discussed my plans and goals for the operation with my longtime associate at Emory Hospital, Dr. Bakay. Then we decided on the surgeon in Belize to handle my brain surgery: Dr. Joel Cervantes at the 'Quality of Life' clinic in Belize City.

---

[9] "On Being" with Krista Tippett. "A conversation with Dr. Atul Gawanda."

On June 21, 2014, Dr. Cervantes conducted a 10-hour operation, successfully implanting multiple Electrodes in the speech motor cortex of my brain, which is just above my left ear. The operation was successful. When I awoke the following morning I was speaking normally and writing clearly.

That afternoon I fell into a deep sleep, optimistic about my recovery, and not anticipating any of the unintended consequences that appeared the next day. On Day 2 when I awoke, I had lost my speech and my ability to write, and felt weak on my right side.

Dr. Cervantes team did a CAT scan on my brain, revealing a significant amount of postoperative edema. This is always a possibility following such a complicated and invasive procedure, but we had no way of knowing the results would be as severe: the swelling had generated so much pressure around the language area of my primary motor cortex that I suddenly found myself profoundly "locked-in," as incapable of normal speech or writing as many of my research subjects had been.

Unable to even pen a short note, I began my recovery in a room in the ICU and watched the World Cup soccer on cable TV. Dr. Cervantes prescribed a course of anti-swelling medications, and after five days I began to get some recovery from my paralysis and speech loss though I still felt fatigued and weak on my right side. At this point, a nurse began helping me through the recovery process, day to day, and we focused on speech and motor exercises, gradually extending the length of the therapy in tandem with the degree of reduced swelling in my brain. By week two, I'd moved across the street to a simple adobe villa, an area of guest rooms for outpatients and rehabilitation. Naturally, as I soldiered through days where I could only speak three or four words, and would spend an hour trying to write a simple sentence, I had plenty of time to reflect on my last year in sessions with Erik Ramsey.

After my initial years of research with Erik, he became more ill and from roughly 2009 to 2012 he stayed home, in between unscheduled visits to the ER. His energy level, concentration and ability to be in the "here and now" fluctuated week-to-week. But in 2013 year nine after his first implant, we began a series of "conditioning sessions," conditioning experiments that allowed him to be more responsive and that supported a return to mapping neural signals. I recorded again with Erik in 2014, quite a few months before my own surgery in Belize, but he was so ill that any movement of his head caused him to pass out. He had fought hard to go forward with the signal mapping, but once again the state of his health rapidly declined, shutting down our decade-long, shared journey.

RETURN VOYAGES

Dr. Cervantes released me when my recovery of normal speech was about 50 percent. I returned to my Neural Signals office in Duluth, and began seeing patients again in my neurological practice. But as the summer ended and the trees above my lab turned from yellow to gold, I decided to return to Belize, as soon as my normal speech had recovered 100 percent. If I did not have the electronic sending components attached to my Electrodes then I could not complete the planned study comparing my audible and silent word formations.

Dr. Cervantes and his team did attach the components, and this time I returned to my lab speech intact, and moved on to several months of recording neural signals. Unfortunately, one area of the scalp incision did not close and heal completely, and 28 days into my neural signal testing, I closed things down on that project. My third and final surgery to remove the just added power coil and transceiver was January 13, 2015. However, I did succeed in decoding silent speech as effectively as audible speech.

Today my perspective on the BCI field is that it is moving too slowly. The cost of development and the difficulty of obtaining funding and leaping through FDA hoops doesn't allow a more sanguine forecast. Even so, we are now just 10 years from Ray Kurzweil's technological singularity, and, concurrently, I believe that the enhancement of human brains will occur with incremental growth in our cognitive and communication abilities. My years working with the BCI candidates prove the concept and still holds promise for future locked-in individuals who want to raise their quality of life and recover their ability to speak and better define their "here and now". We can even now say that JR was the first cyborg! No question about that: He was able to control the computer. I did not reach cyber status -- even though I was implanted -- for I did not control the computer. Erik was also a cyborg within the field of physical brain implants, and he definitely did move the cursor with his neural signals.

Though not always in the spotlight as brain enhancement research, our gains in BCI discoveries allowed me to see two more personal sides of what science and medicine can do. As Dr. Gawande said in BEING MORTAL: "We've been wrong about what our job is in medicine. We think our job is to ensure health and survival. But really, it is larger than that, it is really to enable well-being. And well-being is the reason one wishes to be alive".

To be alive is to communicate. Whether we move ahead with invasive or noninvasive decoding, the speech prosthesis will gradually advance using recent breakthroughs in neural net, deep learning paradigms. This approach gains in power and accuracy the more it is used, an appropriate corollary to the way a child's brain initially develops.

I believe the next decade holds exciting progress in silent brain digitized speech. That "Sea of Darkness" that so many locked-in and paralyzed individuals have suffered through, is finally being explored. The uncharted waters, with those unknown dragons on the edge of the maps, are being transformed from a Sea of Darkness to a Sea of Dreams. And having dreams is a reason to be alive.

I'm grateful for all the brave souls who voyaged along with me. And, you know, those dragons may turn out to be brilliant dolphins, teaching us to speak all over again...

Chapter 9

CONVERSATIONS BETWEEN EDDIE RAMSEY AND PHIL KENNEDY ON JUNE 3ᴿᴰ AND 19ᵀᴴ, 2019

EDDIE RAMSEY

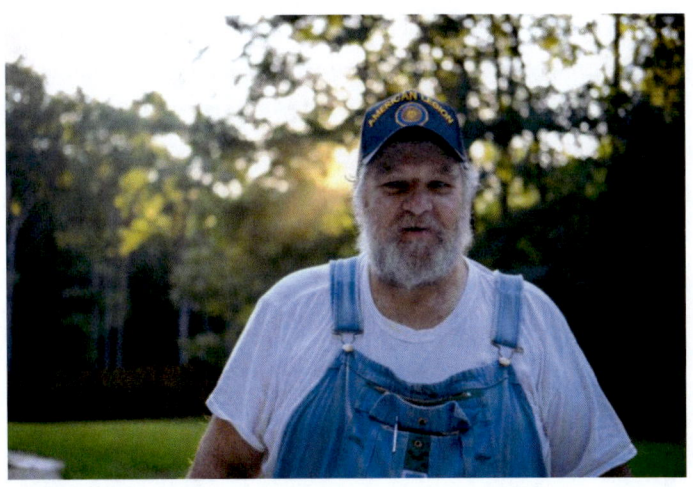

Phil: Erik was 16 years old when he suffered the brainstem stroke and 34 years old when he died, 18 years. That's a chunk of your life. It was very stressful. I remember you always coming into the lab and there always complaining about the insurance companies.

Eddie: The insurance companies always fight you tooth and nail. They don't want to pay for anything and you either have to get two or three doctors to say what you need, or you just say what you need, and it gets submitted and it goes to a committee. Even with two or three doctors it can still go to a committee for approval. And what I find works the best is to make it work to their advantage. For the $5,000 mattress that we eventually got, I said listen, you are not treating him for bedsores because he doesn't have any. We have to have a plastic cover over the mattress because he is quadriplegic, his catheter comes off, so we have to make sure he has no dermal breakdown. It took me more than four years to get the bed.

One thing that didn't bother me were the people at Sheppard Center – they were fabulous – they helped me get the overhead lift. It was new and it's a railing on the ceiling and you can move the person from the bed to the wheelchair and vice versa. It worked great. You wouldn't believe how many families I talked to about needing one and none of them got theirs approved.

P: They knew the angle.

E: They knew the angle alright.

P: So how does endlessly battling like that feel now?

E: My take on life is: Things are meant to be. They happen, you know. There is nothing you can do to change. If you were meant to die on a train wreck or whatever and somehow it got averted, in a couple of weeks or months, it would happened again. I pretty much believe life is pre-planned.

P: So you believe in predestination. I don't really believe in it. Let's say you are a reckless driver and you will crash and die. So you can change to being a safe driver and avert that, right?

E: But then you have that dare devil Evil Kinevel when all he did was keep crashing, more than most any motorcyclists there was.

P: Did he eventually die?

E: Yes, but I think it was from natural causes. But maybe from complications of broken bones. What I am getting at is, you are dealt a hand and either you play that hand or you fold. Erik was 16 years old when he became locked-in.

P: Gosh, my son Nash has just turned 15. Like you say it just happens. You either give up or you fought it. So you fought it. Very good!

E: The way you and I interacted in Erik's case, I had just run out of options for him to communicate, and that was something he had to have.

P: You heard about my research at medical school.

E: Right.

P: They knew about it. We were chatting about options. I remember you came around we started chatting about possibilities. I would like to give you the seven chapters to read because he (Brian Shaw) really lays on what we were facing. I wrote answers to these questions. He asked me the tough questions. I had to dig into myself to answer them. I am sure you've experienced similar moments.

E: I think my only regret is that I got worn down after a while and eventually let the doctors dictate his treatment. [tearful]. When he got "pneumonia", it didn't manifest like they said. They kept saying "pneumonia" in his left lung, but actually he had that scar tissue and they kept diagnosing that as pneumonia.

P: That was stupid.

E: I put it in the record. Anyway, after a while, I didn't take such good care of him as I did, to make him go through hell, what was happening, so he could enjoy life as well as he could. And when they told me he *had* to have the tracheotomy that was when he started going downhill. [tearful].

P: They were wrong. When he was coming in here he did not have the trach.

E: Yes, he just had the scaring. They took the button out in Sheppard so he could clear his throat. So think about it: we kept him for 14 or 15 years without it. I think it was longer than that. I would rather just have him pass away than not having him breath.

P: His stroke extended. His brainstem got more involved and that is why his blood pressure was out of control. I was talking to a friend of mine, Thomas Wichmann, he had done work on the first patient. He asked if he got Wallerian degeneration, and I told him he got more than that. Wallerian degeneration is post stroke degeneration of the long axons that you can see on MRI, clearly. I said Thom (Phil's friend), at the end, he lost control of his autonomic control system, so if you lifted his head he would pass out. So he lay flat all the time. Thom said that is why the trach and vent were needed. It was terrible.

E: It wears on you having to fight for everything. If it wasn't the insurance companies, it was the government, because they endlessly ask for more and more data. To give them everything, it feels you must have a law degree and be a doctor. Because usually you haven't a clue. You gave me direction on much of it.

P: I remember one question Brian asked that is still food for thought: The first hour in ER Erik thrashes around, talked and screamed in pain. He wasn't locked-in. So what made him locked-in? It must have been tough at first wondering if he had a stroke or not. He was moving around ...

E: He was talking. He was moving, asking for ice chips, screaming in pain, when he went into surgery, 24 hours later, he was lethargic in the bed. The doctor kept coming in rubbing his feet with a sharp object, seeing if he get a reaction. But only moving his eyes was all they could see.

P: Your family and friends came around.

E: They helped a lot. [tearful].

P: It does yeah, so essential.

E: Those first years, his best friend helped out, he would come by the house. He would talk to Erik for hours on end.

P: Erik would give his eye blinks?

E: Erik would laugh at times, just move. He understood everything Mike was saying. He was just carrying on. Basically, Erik would get tickled at certain points. Mike had to get on with his life. He got married, had children, but for about near 3 years, he was over with Erik constantly talking with him. That was a fine friend.

P: I will tell you, what disappointed me is that we did not eventually get him speaking. He did a lot though.

I was thinking about what am I going to do now. There were several issues. One was that we did not have enough signals. We will try to get hundreds of signals in the next patient. And the other thing was Erik could never speak, but we figured out ways to get him to speak. I used the neural net programs in Matlab. 10 years ago it was just beginning. So we had a control period and then speaking audibly and silently, and compared the three sets of data. I realized that, from working with Erik that is something we need to do. It worked out. That is big, really big. So, knowing that, it's the way we'd do it now.

E: You know, when we first came over and we talked about an implant. I was really interested in doing an implant on me at the same time. But the FDA would not approve that. It would have sped up the research immensely. I would be able to communicate. We would have been able to compare my data with Erik's. We would have had a baseline to use.

P: Yes, in one sense, except that everybody is different. It would have given us a control; I had that in my implantation. During silent speech the neural activity was similar as during audible speech.

E: When you were doing the research on yourself, did you try the humming and singing?

P: I never got around to it.

E: Oh okay ...

P: When I put the Electrodes in, we then put the electronics in three months later but I did not want them. I wanted to externalize the Electrodes. I built the Electrodes with bulky connectors, so when you cut the scalp over them they would be pointing up. So then we had to connect the single channels so we could only put in three and the incision started to break down. I kept it clean so when the surgeon wanted to take it out, I said no, not yet, so "just sew it up". So we kept doing that for weeks while I collected data and we got away with it. So I got the phrases, the words and phones and sensory. That wasn't bad. I got a lot, but I didn't do any humming or singing.

I will tell you one thing about Erik. When we went back and did the conditioning study at year nine. Years before we presented Erik with tones and a guitar sound resulted in one unit firing like crazy, like nuts. About five years later we went back and presented the same guitar sound and the same unit fired like crazy.

E: Did we ever leave the computer on when Erik was listening to his music? Just let him listen to music.

P: I don't think we recorded that. He would have been responding to Slipknot.

E: He really would.

P: I still have those. Do you want them?

E: I guess so. My granddaughter loves Slipknot.

P: We have a bunch of other CDs left over from the project. It was quite a saga.

E: I was really glad we ran into you and you were doing this crucial research. I didn't know how to occupy his life. He looked forward to coming down to the lab.

P: I remember one time, in an interview, you said it would give him something to do. And that is true. I did not take that badly.

E: You can only watch several thousands of movies before getting bored, and no matter how much you like Slipknot, 365 days of it is a bit much.

P: I remember at the end, at the funeral, I was so upset. I made a complete fool of myself. I was crying.

E: You did great.

P: I consider life to be so precious. That is why I am so against abortion. Any life. You know. I am not talking about vegetative states here. But someone like Erik who is aware, smart, there is someone living in there.

E: So long as he wasn't in pain, and as long as I could give him something to keep him occupied so he doesn't get bored.

P: I remember my early years when I worked in neurosurgery, people would come in as a quadriplegic, the resident would go down to the parents and ask 'what do you want to do'. He explained the situation, showed there was no hope for recovery. So they just turned it (the ventilator) off. I understand why they would. I get that. But I am really determined to get this out. Let me tell you what we are going to do. We are doing new work with a company who implant electronics. They have one for recording EMG channels. So I am working with them to modify their system, 16 bipolar channels, high bandwidth and they use infrared for transmission, not FM. So we are trying to get that going and use that to implant more patients. SBIR, 2 years and god knows how many years to get through the FDA. You go through so much....

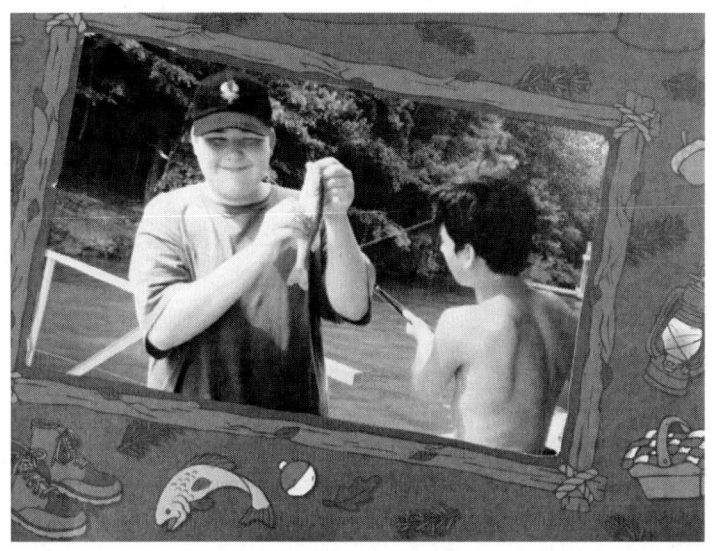

What I am going to do is use the "pedestal" component like everyone else. It goes through the scalp. It avoids the implanted electronics because it allows a connection to the Electrode wires by connecting onto the pedestal from the outside. Blackrockmicro Inc sell it. I asked them to sell it without the Utah array. You know the Utah array – it breaks down after a few years, 85 percent loss after 3 years. So I said no. (They said) I have to sell it to you with the Utah array. $6750 for one. You have to have two for surgery. I discussed it with the rep and he says he has a few that are not meeting criteria. He will sell them cheap. That would mean using the pedestal and implanting more people.

You remember Chad Gambrell? He is the computer programmer. I am talking to Chad about modifying a program he wrote. He writes software and he says it will work as well as Matlab's. Otherwise we have to pay for Matlab.

So we are looking to find more people. Not yet FDA approved. The FDA, my best friends.

E: I know the relationship! [Laughs]

P: So we will go back to where we went before, to Belize. No reason not to go again. Bring them back here into the lab. Let me tell you, we would not have gone this far if it were not for Erik. Coming in 2 to 3 days per week, very slow, like watching paint dry. I got that.

E: [Laughs]

P: Jon Brumberg got a PhD out of it. I was on his committee. I actually nailed him a little bit. For a PhD you have to make an original contribution to knowledge, and aaah, he answered very well. He got it anyway!

E: The session Erik enjoyed most was when he moved the cursor. Frank Guenther, Jon Brumberg, Meel Velliste were all there.

P: They got excited when Erik moved the cursor. I still have that video. Its part of the book.

E: But on the flip side, was that last year when he became immobile. [tearful]. He could hardly breath. On the vent. Trouble breathing. Congestion was worse.

P: Did he ever express to you his goal?

E: The only time we had communication was when he was in the emergency room, and then we had the board with alphabet. He used the board to display his sense of humor, like getting the caregiver to look for something that did not exist! [Laughs].

P: Did his brothers help out?

P: How about the wrestler? What was his name?

E: That was Joseph. He was friend of the family for quite a few years. He was his caregiver. As far as his brothers were concerned. When they were over, it was a relief to me. His older brother took him to rock concerts, to legacy football, Falcons training camp. When the Falcons gave Erik free passes to games, they went there. Braves games also. They took him a lot of places, usually once or twice per month. Chris knew more about what was going on, he knew what Erik liked. Matt (younger brother) liked skateboarding and stuff, and Erik roller-bladed. They had different friends. Chris was off the middle of the day and was either at school or going to tech school in NC and was able to help out a lot. They would give him food. Everybody was trained to make sure the whole family knew to feed him, bath him. The biggest thing I was worried about was skin breakdown. I had an aunt who had skin breakdown. They used sheepskins and the complications...

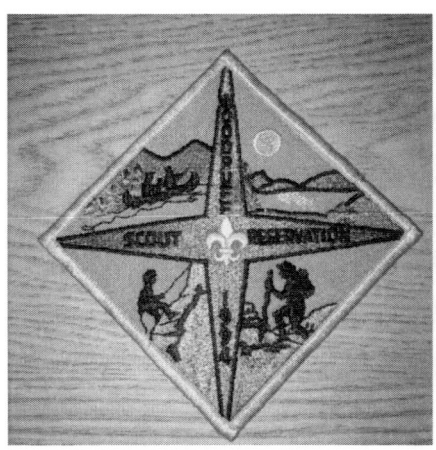 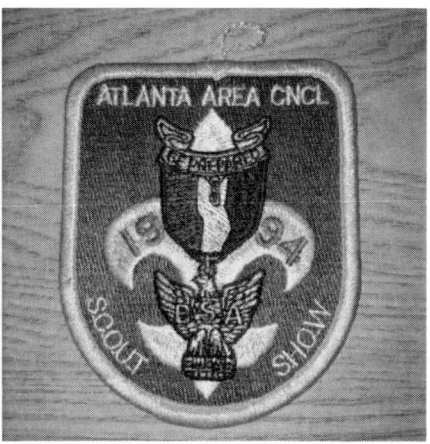

Erik's boy scout badges.

E: But, big picture, he was never able to let me know what he wanted. That was the most frustrating thing for him because even with the 'yes' and 'no' eye movements, sometimes it was hard for him to indicate, sometimes 'yes', sometimes 'no'.

P: I had to often ask you what did he say. [laughs]

E: I never really got a specific goal, but I am sure that communicating was one. If he was able to communicate in any way that was consistent we would have been able to get more out of it.

P: He could not accurately control his eyes, yet there are systems that use eye movements. It is very slow, not like speaking. He could not even look straight, he had to look at the wall where we projected images, he had to look to the side. He could not foveate it.

E: Did the grants pay for his research?

P: They paid earlier on, paying for his implantation. So then we just did it with the folks here, Jesse and Steven Seibert and then Joe Wright. Thin crowd now. I have a student, a very smart student. We are still analyzing his data as well as mine. We will publish it again.

E: When you were doing the phones, did each one have their own signature of signals?

P: Yes. That is a question we want to answer again with Matlab. There is a Classification app there and it takes all the phones and see how well they differ from one another.

E: All right.

P: That is what I still want to do. We never did enough words with Erik. That's what we want to reanalyze.

P: Oh I did not tell you. We took a piece of brain where the Electrode lay, we took it to Marla Gearin in Emory and did the whole histology. It was wonderful. No scarring after 13 years in the brain. I was able to see the piece of tissue and slide the wires out of the tissue. So she took a section every 100 microns and stained for the scarring, for myelination, neurafilaments. So it is sent for publication. It was wonderful, awesome. Thank you for letting me do that. So we can connect the recordings to the underlying tissue and make it more convincing. We see the neurites. We also see the oval holes in the tissue where we saw three and then one (wire).

E: The only time we saw those wires, on an X-ray or a CT scan.

P: But this tissue evaluation confirms everything. We grow the tissue inside the Electrode.[laughs].

E: I never regretted doing the research, never. It gave Erik's life some true meaning.

P: He was the first person in whom we tried to restore continuous speech. The first person. We succeeded in understanding how to do it. We did not have the Matlab apps in 2008 and now they are there. It is phenomenal. It encourages me to go on to the next case.

E: Well good luck. I am all for it. If you want me to talk to any prospective parents, a patient, whatever, I would be happy to.

P: Awesome. That would be great. Thanks Eddie. The other thing is David Burke is coming over in July or August and he will want us to chat again. Bring his camera and all that carry on…

E: I will see if I can get some new overalls. My wife says will you please wear your best clothes. I told her Dr. Kennedy is used to me wearing my overalls.

P: I know the Falcons were high on Erik's sports list … Any good stories? Sneaked in without tickets, maybe?

E: They may have before the accident.

P: Your boys all got free tickets, right?

E: They did get free tickets.

P: How did they wrangle those?

E: I wrote to Mike Smith, the Falcon's coach, and I explained to him Erik's situation. The office up there sent us a package of 10 tickets, press passes, field passes, the works. Even met a bunch of cheerleaders.

P: I am sure he liked that.

E: Oh, yeah, I forget which game we went to, but we sat right above the tunnel where they come out and the thing is we had our choice of front row or on the field, but we could not get in there (with Erik's wheelchair) and I explained that so Mike put us on the first mezzanine, which is only 10 or 12 feet back. The next person's head was below Erik's feet so I mean he could see the whole field. His brothers enjoyed it too, they got signatures from Falcon quarterback Matt Ryan: and I'm sure there were some 'sign here for my brother' too.

Another thing: we went up there before the season started. All the linemen knew about Erik so they made him an honorary Offensive Linemen. They all had beards, some had red hair, so he fit right in with them.

P: That's great. So did he go to many practices?

E: For 5 or 6 years in a row, we went to every practice they had. He got to know a lot of Falcon players! Same thing with the Braves but they didn't send us any tickets. We went probably to 10 or 12 Braves games.

P: But they never gave you any free tickets – and look what happened to them! Bad Karma.

E: We took him to several Legacy Football games. He really enjoyed them. Of course, you have half-naked women running up and down the field. Actually, man, they make them wear these shorts with garters on them. The garters are just hanging there. And they wear short tops. They wear rugby pads, shoulder pads and rugby helmets. They wear knee pads. Several of the girls got injured really bad. We also went to one of those arena games. It was way up in Gwinnett county.

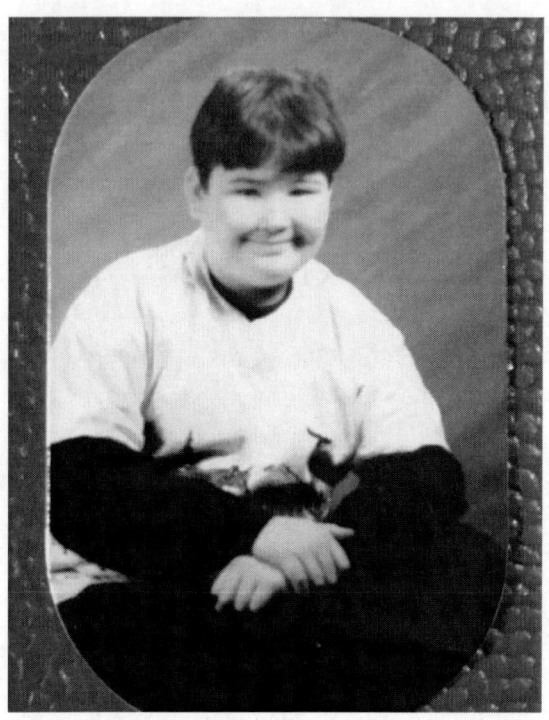

P: The arena surface is not as good, as soft, as grass. So they hit the wall and everything.

E: One of the girls hit the wall and flipped over. There were five guys there willing to grab her and send her back!

Several wrestling matches were on his radar. WWF sent him a lot of free passes. He enjoyed it, or his brothers enjoyed it and they dragged him along. When they dragged him along he never complained.

P: (Laugh)

E: I remember an enormous hard rock concert, took place up at Gwinnett civic center. Chris even took off work that day, and the concert was free outside. Several bands were playing in the evening. Chris and I took Erik up there during the day. There were like five tractor trailers, with bands playing. The had stands with tons of mementos to buy, and they were even giving away lots of stuff. Erik made a huge haul that day.

Do you know the guy in California who sent Erik the CDs?

P: I do. I remember him.

E: He sent Erik well over 2,000 CDs! Did you know that?

P: Oh really?

E: 2,000 hard-rock CDs. There were bands from everywhere. And he even snuck in five Slipknot CDs.

P: Who was he?

E: He was a producer out in California. I think he read an article, and he called you and asked if he could send CDs. You said sure. That meant a lot to Erik. Almost unlimited listening time to his favorite genre of music and his favorite band.

When I got all the CDs it was an enormous box. $50 or $60 just to ship it. We constantly played them, wore out one CD player and had to buy another one. Erik never got tired of listening to them. Many were bands people had never heard of at the time, but now they are bands people know well.

P: They were just starting out.

E: You know, I liked hard rock when I was over in Europe with the Air Force. Listened to it all the time with Erik and he thought it was kind of neat that I would listen to hard rock.

P: Great….. Had Erik begun driving before his accident? Started dating?

E: I went and got him a manual to read. A week later he said he would take his driver test. I asked him did you read that book? No, but he said he knew everything there was to know about driving. He failed miserably.

P: OK

E: It wasn't but a few months after that he had the accident. So he wasn't dating anyone with a car, but I know that a lot of girls at school from all the teachers' conferences, and Erik attracted a lot of young ladies because of his graphic art.

P: He was a funny guy, right?

E: He was then. He liked to draw animated pornography and the girls were curious and fascinated.

P: Really?

E: So I know a lot of young girls liked him, and everything, and …

P: Beware

E: The only girl from his class I knew, was there when he came out of surgery. This was a young girl, her hair dyed blue, she came and saw him, broke down in tears and then she never returned. I tried to find out who it was, but no one could tell me. A young girl with black hair dyed blue? 200 girls in high school? But everyone in school came to see him for a while. The ICU was packed. The nurse told me we could not have that many people in the waiting room. They wouldn't let them stay long. He also had quite a few teachers visit. They were trying to find out if they could teach him at the hospital, what arrangements could be made. I told them that until we found out something else, there was no point. He was in ICU a whole 30 days, before the Shepherd Center.

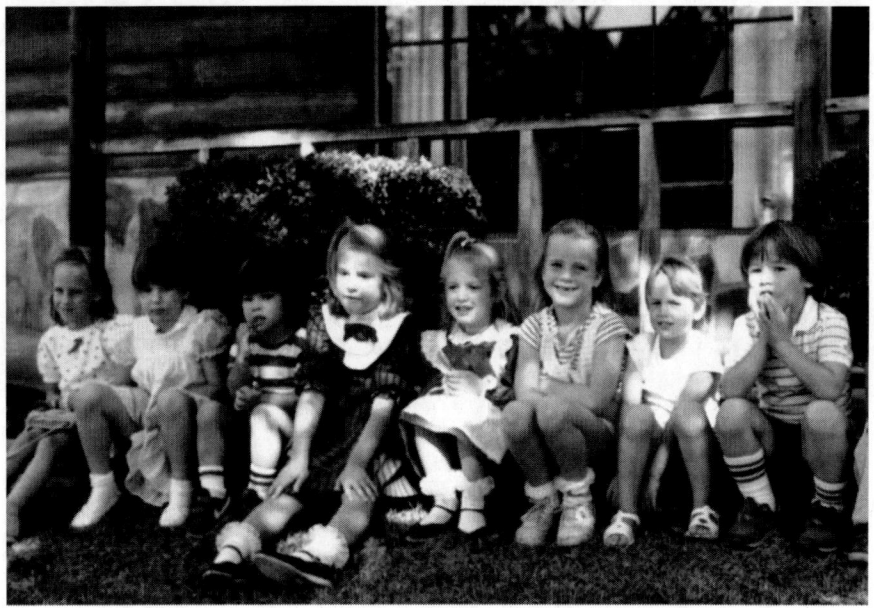

Erik, at right, always had lots of girlfriends!

P: Did he have a special teacher there?

E: She was a special ed teacher over at Berkmar. There was her and two or three people in Gwinnett that came and tried different methods, different switches, to see if he could push a switch with a finger. Actually, there was one he could do sometimes with his thumb. But the speech therapist at the

Shepherd Center said that unless it is repetitive and on command, and do it at least 80% of the time, it is not worth pursuing from a teaching standpoint.

P: So it was at this point that you introduce the letter board?

E: That's right. I set up the letter board system for him. This was when the speech therapist was trying all the different buttons, eye movements, and so on. I don't know why I came up with the letter board. She was talking about his eye movement, up for 'yes' and down for 'no'. He was going through some depression, so when I found out he could do 'yes' and 'no', we can go through the alphabet. It worked sometimes and after a year and a half he lost interest. I don't know what happened. They think that the pneumonia caused something in the brain to atrophy. I think he lost interest in it. At one point I was fairly fast with it and he was too, and I would start guessing the words, and he wasn't real happy with that. (laughs). He wanted to spell out everything for the sense of accomplishment it gave him.

The one good time he had with the letter board he was trying to get the caregiver to try and find that movie. When I got home from work, she had broken English and some Spanish, she asked "can you find this movie?" She was very attentive and she tried to keep him happy, so I looked at him and said "I can't figure this out". So I did it again. It made a little more sense but it did not completely match the other title. So I am thinking, how can the title be: "bees are purple". What movie is that? Right!

P: (Laughs)

E: Is this thing a movie? We wondered ....? He just died laughing (in his own way)! I said "You had her looking for a movie all day?" He indicated "yes". And he started laughing. He still had that warped sense of humor.

P: (Laugh)

E: She was real sweet.

P: So he was well able to tease everybody. I am sure he wanted some kind of control.

We have mentioned his stint at the Shepherd Center. So any Shepherd stories?

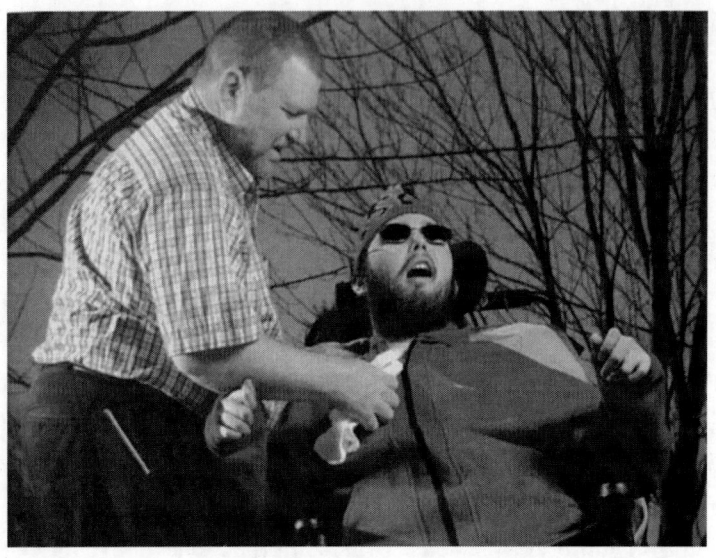

Erik Laughing!

E: Yeah, there are lots of Shepherd stories! He was in ICU in Gwinnett for 30 days. They were talking about putting him in a nursing home or rehabilitation. I had no doubt in my mind we were going to care for him. So we needed to go and get trained and evaluate him. So they gave us Scottish Rite, Shepard and another one. The third one was for elderly people. The Scottish Rite, when we went over there, most of the children were under 15 and teenagers, a lot of them had cancer. To us it was kind of depressing. As young as they were, he liked children but we thought it would be better if he could communicate with people his age.

P: Shepherd was the best, then?

E: To us, it was the only choice. The thing was, we roll in there in the ambulance, the doctor and five people come out and just ignored Sandra and me. They take him upstairs to evaluate him, and they are sitting there talking. I forget the doctor's name. But the nurse said, " Lousy bedside manner, but he is the best doctor in this whole hospital." And he was too.

The first thing he did was to remove all five of Erik's IVs, and then he took all his medicines, put them in a box, and said "no more medications". When we left Gwinnett Medical Center, all the things that were keeping him alive were being taken away!

P: Really?

E: So what they did was they put him on the water bed, they gave him an IV with saline so he did not dehydrate. And they asked what formula was he on. I said I did not know. So he said it does not matter anyway. So the doctor recommended what he wanted to start him on. Then they said does he like anything. We said yes he loves sweet tea. And they said "oooh". We will give him sweet tea but not right now. We will wait three or four weeks. They will evaluate his swallowing. We will put him on recreational feeding and give him things that he can swallow. I said okay.

P: He was on the vent at that time?

E: He was on the vent in Gwinnett. So one of the first things they did was to get him the speech therapist, the physical therapist, the dietitian, the occupational therapist, I forget but they were all specialists in their fields. So the doctor came in and talked to Sandra and I, this is where he was, this is what we think is going on, and this is where we are going from here. Which one of you will be here 24 hours a day, for the next 30 days and I said I am. So I took off work, using my annual leave from work. I stayed there 24 hours a day for 30 days.

P: You mean you slept there?

E: Oh, yes! Slept there, I ate there. What they wanted was someone to learn the whole routine, and they wanted it to be a family member if he was going to stay at home. If not they wanted to put him in assisted living or a nursing home. They said if one family member is willing to commit to keeping him alive, we will train them. So I was there for every physical therapy session, occupational therapy. The thing is they show you once, and that's it, you do it every time. He had drop foot and they put a cast and gradually put pressure on it every five days, until we got it better. Along with range of motion exercises, I was there for every speech therapy session, we tried every button, every switch. I learned how to dress him, change his diaper, change his catheter, I learned how to take care of his trach. I learned how to groom him, brush his teeth without swallowing his tooth brush. They teach you everything from the ground up.

P: Impressive.

E: They even give you a 3 inch binder and you learn everything. If I were to learn this in college going to my classes, I would never have gotten through it. Everything that's in there, you have to learn. They are so efficient. And if you have any hopes about miracles, they tell you go to the preacher and talk to him. They deal with you strictly on the medical end.

P: Right.

E: They said, "we are not trying to downplay miracles, we believe in miracles, but we **don't** do miracles here". They **didn't** want to build a false hope.

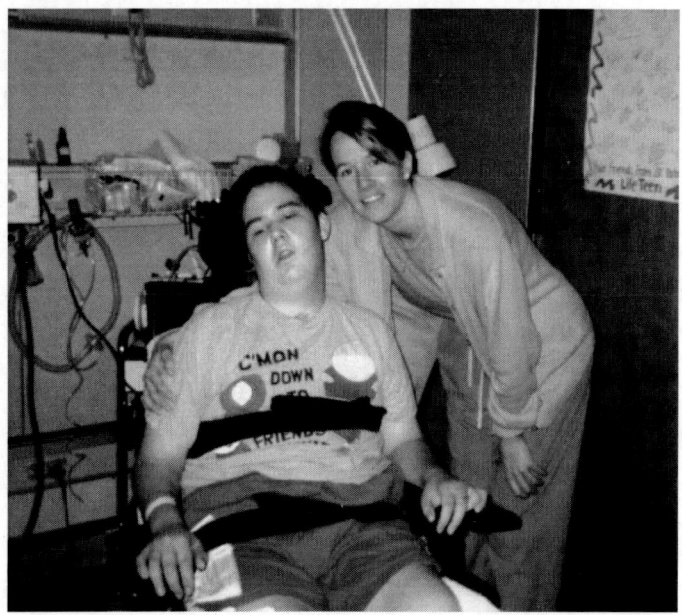

Erik with Sheppard Center nurse

P: Exactly.

E: And the other thing was, they knew Erik was quadriplegic, but they kept the rails up on the side of his bed. They said they have people who are unconscious and wake up, and get up and fall and bust their head open because they had no rails up. But, when they took the trach out, there are three things, the trach, the button and a third thing not sure what it was. Once they found out his cough reflex was strong, the doctor kept asking the nurse

"How is his cough reflex"? Every time he walked into the room he would ask. And when I would answer, he would say "OK" and he was looking for more than I could offer. Once he found his cough reflex was good, and he could clear his throat if something got lodged in his throat on his own, that was when he decided to take the button off (his trach opening) before he went home.

P: Right.

E: After three weeks they allowed him to have his sweet tea, mixed with corn starch.

P: To thicken it up?

E: Yeah, to thicken it up. But we cheated! We took the corn starch out, used the straw and only let him have small amounts.

P: I seem to remember you guys were giving him some food to eat as well.

E: We cheated a lot.

P: No kidding!

E: They did wheelchair analysis there. What type of wheelchair would be suitable for him. I didn't know there were that many wheelchairs. They decided to start out with a manual wheelchair. Shepherd helped us find the wheelchair. We got a beach wheelchair and I had to pay for that. The insurance company looked at it and disapproved it because we did not live at the beach. But we did use it to walk in the park. They helped with the overhead lift and that overhead was the greatest thing. So many people had been turned down for that not even the doctors could believe we got it.

P: How much did they pay for it?

E: I have no idea. All I know is the doctor maybe did not have a good bedside manner and someone you would not want to get into a casual conversation with, but he liked treating patients. He liked being good at what he did. He did not like insurance companies. He just had ordered lifts for the hospitals, made in Sweden or somewhere like that. They were incredibly expensive: Rails and fancy stuff. They got them in about half the rooms in Shepherd.

P: You got one at home?

E: We got the very expensive one, the "Mercedes" one, out of the models available. The other thing was we did not know how to order the rails because there were straight and curved sections. The curved ones could be a quarter or an eight of a circle? This is aircraft grade aluminum! He ordered 10 of the curved and 10 of the straight rails for us. We had enough to furnish the whole hospital.

P: He ordered so many for the hospital?

E: No, he ordered those for us!

P: Seriously?

E: They approved the whole lot!

P: He has some magic.

E: The thing was we only used two sections of the straight rails and four of the curved rails. So we used only six sections out of the twenty! When I realized that I called the doctor and said we got too much rail. "Keep it," he said. "Don't tell me or them you got too much. The trick is if they approve something, don't tell them that you screwed up. They approved something and if you say it's too much, the next time they will fight you tooth and nail for whatever else you want." So we kept all the extra rails.

The thing was when we moved to Buford, the technician came to mount the rails on the ceiling, he came up there and asked why we have so much extra rails? You know how much this costs? And I said I know what it cost 20 years ago (when Eddie was in the Air Force). And I said I'll trade it to you for moving the system and mounting it on the ceiling. And he said fine with me! So we got the system moved for free.

P: Are you serious?

E: Sure. Apparently, he was going to make some really good money out of that rail.

P: That's awesome.

E: I didn't care. The main thing I wanted was to get it to work.

P: So did Sandra have any stories about him? I know you were the main guy.

E: She probably does. She buried herself in work. We were married for many years and she always worked. But I have never seen her dive into her work like she did when Erik got sick. I asked her if she had anything to say, and she said she had nothing to add.

P: I mean I can imagine her distress and your distress. Men are different. You know, we have a problem and we feel down and them get mad at it and go fix the problem.

E: Yeah.

P: I guess she just dived into her work. A not-for-profit. A very good thing to do. It gave her great satisfaction.

E: She was still the boss of the family! If something was not getting done it should get done, she would straighten us all out and tell us the new rules of the day.

P: A true woman.

E: That's great. The one other thing that happened in Shepherd was I had to go home and take a shower. They only want their patients taking showers. I had to go home and take a shower, got changed and got something to eat and went back. When I got back he was sitting in his wheelchair in the hallway and he was crying.

P: Really?

E: Because I had left and he missed me. [Eddie cries].

P: Thanks for sharing that with us. You are a tremendous example to any other parents with a tragedy like that. You just got to go and do what you can. Don't expect miracles. But if you think of the life hereafter, he is up there and you are going straight up Eddie.

E: (loud laughter). Chris his brother, and a good friend of his, Christine, she came over to see Erik. It was funny. She was leaning on the rail. He couldn't turn his head except sometimes, but he was able to turn his head that night. He was talking to her. She said "after a while, I looked at his eyes, and you know he couldn't move his eyes left and right", we said yeah, "well he could surely look down my blouse."

P: Really?

E: After she figured it out and he turned his head sideways, she said, "did you enjoy the free show?" Times like that, you know, you could tell when he was having a good day. He would "laugh."

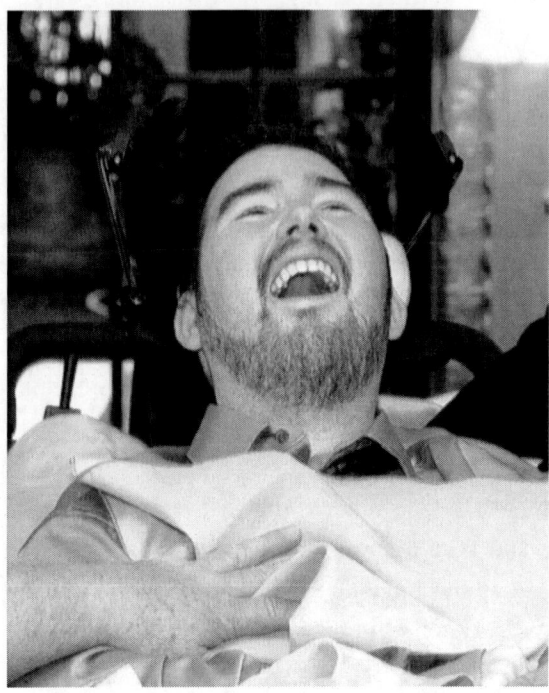

Sometimes he would "connect" with people he liked: Like Donna, his third or fourth caregiver. She was from Columbia and a physical therapist. And she was real cute girl, roughly about the same age as Erik. She stayed in the house and slept in the room with him. She loved to watch the Simpsons, and if Erik was able to talk he would have said he liked it anyway since she was so cute. He really enjoyed her as the caregiver. After about a year she drifted away. Now she is a nurse.

P: She was a physical therapist.

E: We all went to his graduation. What was her name, from Columbia, she was walking out in the field and he got the most applause of anybody. Not sure if it was him or her! Everybody knew Erik at Berkmar school.

And he had a caregiver during the day at Berkmar. She was only with him from the time he went to school to the time her got home. She was the school nurse. She could give injections. She stopped them sending Erik to Gwinnett Medical center every five minutes. They were so paranoid about him getting pneumonia. She was a really good nurse. She wore short skirts and everything. She was petite and they thought she was a student there, so she got cafeteria food at a lower price.

P: That's cute.

E: When we went on vacation, one year to Pennsylvania, other years to Philadelphia, Virginia, New York city and Washington DC. When we got to New York city it was really nice. They took him up the freight elevator of the Empire State building. When we got up there the security police cleared off the whole observation deck and we got to walk him around the building.

P: Did you fly or drive?

E: We drove in the van with everyone together. When we would go on vacation everybody would pick a city they would like to visit. For example, my youngest son Matt went to the park in Philadelphia where all the skate boarders were. So we did that and we went to where the constitution was written. From there we went to New York and his brothers wanted their picture taken (with Erik) at the WWE, and then we went to the wax museum. It was after 911, so there was nothing but cardboard wall all around (the twin towers location). We went to DC and mainly went to monuments, memorials, the Wall, Smithsonian exhibits. We went to Williamsburg but it had been raining. Williamsburg is specially well set up for wheelchairs ...

P: Especially in the rain.

E: Yeah. Then we went on a barge across the river to Jamestown and he enjoyed the boat ride. From there we came home.

The cruise we went on, he enjoyed. I think it was mainly because of the women in their bikinis. It was limited where he and I could go because the elevators are not set up for wheelchairs especially an extended wheelchair like his. I would have to take his feet off the cradle and put them down on the floor. He didn't like when his feet are dangling. So we took the elevator to the pool. So we put him in the corner next to the ice cream machine and he would watch the girls go by.

P: I remember you showed me photographs of that when you went there. They got him into the pool.

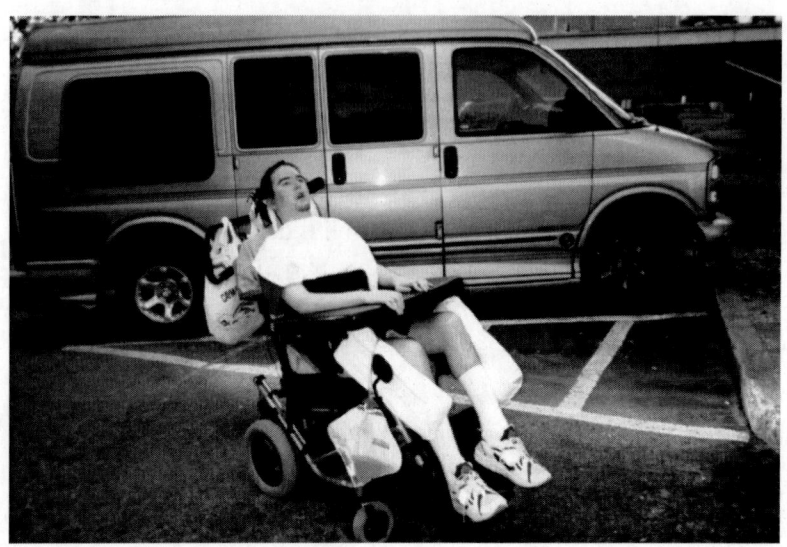

Erik with the travelling van.

E: Yeah. We had ship's officer, an engineer and six or eight crew members, and probably 20 or 30 other people, probably passengers, who just wanted to help.

P: Ah, that's nice.

E: He enjoyed it after he got in there and he knew he wasn't going to sink. He was attached to the cradle and could only go down so far.

P: Attached to the cradle?

E: He sat in the sling, and so he could only go down so far. That's what the engineer was there for. He had an electric motor to lower him.

P: That was real scary for him (Erik).

E: By the time he got in there he was fine. We didn't leave him in there for long.

P: You are one in a million. I think a lot of people would decide to send him to a nursing home.

E: It can be very tough day-to-day: I mean when you think of Christopher Reeves, for all the money he had, he still died from bedsores.

P: Right. We are all so vulnerable.

E: I asked Chris and Matt if they have any stories. But they don't want to tell, so they must be pretty good stories!

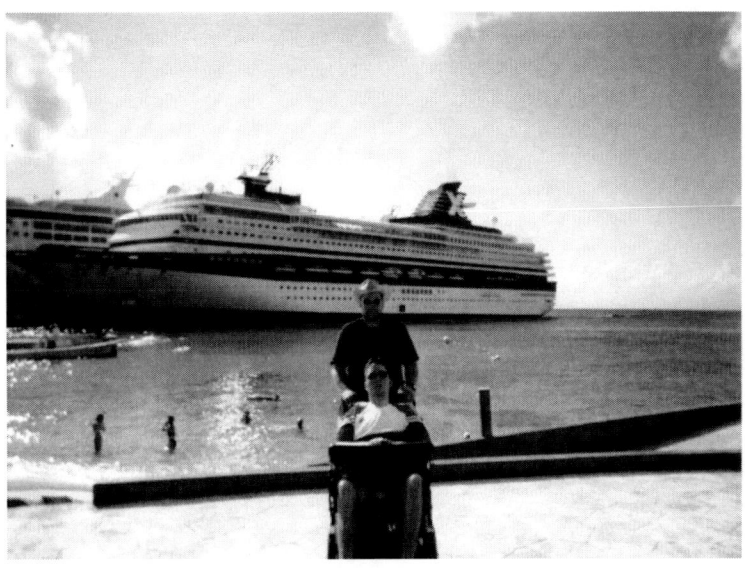

Erik and Eddie before boarding the cruise ship.

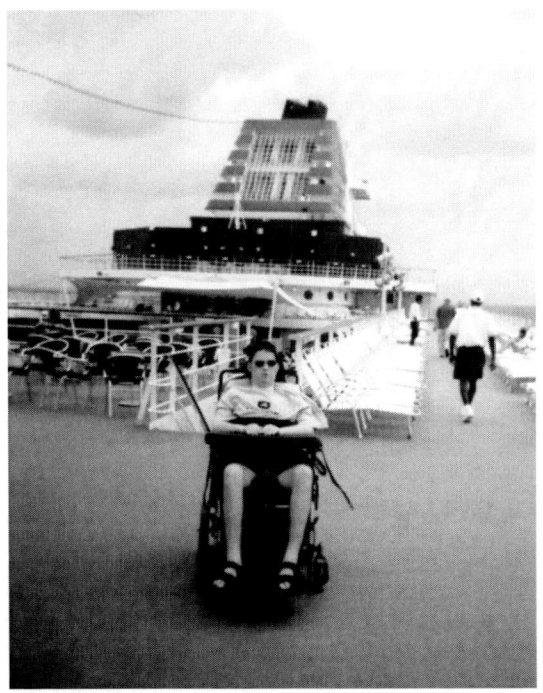

Erik on the cruise ship.

PART 2:
THE SCIENCE BEHIND UNLOCKING ERIK

Chapter 10

INTRODUCTION: "THE INCONVENIENT DETAILS OF LOCKED-IN SYNDROME"

If you are "locked-in" (in the neurological sense of this phrase), you are completely paralyzed and unable to speak, even though you are alert and intelligent and aware of what is going on around you because you can see, hear and smell. The locked-in syndrome is largely due to two conditions. In the first, brainstem stroke suddenly cuts off the information between your body and your brain, thus plunging you into this dreaded state. In the other, ALS more slowly introduces you to your fate. The initials ALS stand for Amyotrophic Lateral Sclerosis, so-called because the motor neurons in the lateral part of the spinal cord undergo a slow death, leading to muscle loss. This results in paralysis that worsens over several years. It is also called Motor Neuron Disease or Lou Gehrig's disease. Gehrig was a beloved baseball player who lost his strength gradually, and so the disease was given his name. A dubious honor!

ALS has no cure but its progress can be slowed down with medications. As the disease ascends into the brainstem and brain, speech is gradually lost and breathing becomes more labored. At this stage a ventilator is required to maintain breathing. Ninety percent of ALS people refuse the ventilator and so accept death. Well known exceptions include the recently deceased

Stephen Hawking who lived more than 50 years on a ventilator and became one the world's most prominent astrophysicists, introducing the concept of Black Holes in space and expanding on Einstein's Theory of Relativity. So all is not lost for those with ALS. However, he is the exception because his disease did not affect his 'thinking' brain. In 50% of people suffering from ALS, the disease affects the 'thinking' part of the brain, and in about 20% of cases it causes a fronto-temporal dementia that is quite severe, leading to hallucinations and depression, as well as memory loss. So those with the 'spinal cord only' version do well, such as Stephen Hawking.

Another example of spinal cord-only ALS, and close to my practice, is David Jayne of Georgia, USA, who bravely fought the disease for more than 30 years. In 2003 I asked David if he would prefer that I try to recover his arm and hand strength or try to recover his speech. This is what he slowly typed out for me (using a muscle twitch in his face to activate a switch that activated his computer):

> Dr. Kennedy asked me if I had the choice of either having hand movement restored or nearly spontaneous speech, which would I chose? I said, there is no question, it would be speech! I am a 15 year survivor of ALS [in 2003]. I have been unable to speak or move my limbs in more than a decade. Yes, restored movement in one arm would offer a fair amount of independence, but speech or even nearly spontaneous speech is a much more liberating and powerful ability. I have used an augmentative communication system for ten years. While having the ability to communicate creates tremendous independence, so much is lost emotionally and in quality of life issues when the communication is not spontaneous. As a father of two young children much bonding never transpired.

That is why, in 2003, I decided to try to restore David Jayne's speech. A simple decision. Actually, there were a few scientific reasons too. First, restoring speech should be easier than restoring movement because smooth movement requires sensory feedback which is a complex array of nerve sensors. That seemed like too much work! What? Restore movement *and* sensory feedback. After all, speech feedback is easy: Hearing! As long as the person can hear, feedback is restored. I agree that sensory feedback from the cheeks, tongue and jaws would enhance the auditory feedback, but is not essential. A second issue is how to activate the many paralyzed muscles. That would require development of muscle stimulation systems. Ouch! Another headache. So I am glad David wanted me to restore his speech, and only his speech!

A Decade of Moments

But, now onto Erik, the Atlanta, Georgia, resident with whom I have done the most research.

In early 2004, Mr. Eddie Ramsey called me to tell me about his son Erik. Erik was 16 years old when he suffered a brainstem stroke and you guessed it, became locked-in, able to move only his eyes and unable to speak or move. Erik's personal story is in part one of this book. This part is the science side, tracking his lab sessions. But before we tell about Erik, let me introduce a few issues about how we do the modifications to the body's communication system.

Prior to developing the Neurotrophic eElectrode I had spent many years recording from brain signals in monkeys with tine type Electrodes, Electrodes that are 2 mm thin and insulated pins with only the recording tip exposed. The problem with the tine type is loss of signal after a few hours of recording. We all knew that these types of Electrodes would not last for the lifetime of a patient who needed a neural prosthetic but we were surprised at how short-lived the actual available recording time was. Hence I had my eyes and ears open to find a better solution.

I was reading the work of the researcher Aquayo and his colleagues from Montréal who, in 1981, showed that a sliver of rat sciatic nerve placed in the rat's brain would grow neurites into the nerve. "Neurite" is a generic term for unmyelinated (immature) axons (tiny tendrils that grow out of the neuronal body to communicate with other neurons). Aquayo then demonstrated that the segment of nerve could cross a damaged part of the brain and form a bridge with neurites growing in each end. They then recorded from these ingrown neurites with tine type Electrodes and found that they were electrically active. When I thought about all this excellent work, I realized that the ingrown neurites might be placed in a hollow cone with recording wires inside, which could greatly extend the recording life of the Electrode.

So I placed slivers of sciatic nerve inside tiny glass cones and inserted them into a rat's brain in my research lab at Georgia Tech, in Atlanta. Histological analysis showed that indeed the neurites grew in and formed a bridge through the cone. So my next step was to put a recording wire inside the glass cone along with the nerve sliver. This allowed me to record the electrical activity. I then placed two recording wires inside and recorded better insulated electrical activity. The resulting signals were published in 1989 after I placed the Electrode into the rat barrel cortex. By deflecting the rat's whiskers I could evoke neural activity within the cone and document that it was present only when specific whiskers were activated and no signal was apparent when the whiskers on the opposite side of the rat's face were activated. This was an Ah-Ah moment for me! After the rat survived for their natural lifetime with no change in the neural activity and continued relationship to the same whiskers, I realized that this could be the basis of a longtime prosthetic device for humans.

I thought every scientist would be delighted with this finding. But nobody seemed to care about it! This was disappointing. So the next thing I did was to implant monkeys in the motor cortex. Together with the late neurosurgeon, Dr. Roy Bakay, I showed that when the monkey moved his arm and made grasping movements different neural signals could be recorded. Furthermore we showed that histological analysis of the tissue inside the glass cone confirmed the ingrowth of neurites. These results were published in the early 1990s [7][10]. Again, nobody seemed very excited about this except Dr. Bakay and myself, with a few exceptions: When we presented these data at a Society for Neuroscience annual meeting, the

---

[10] These data present the histological analysis of the tissue inside the cone tip, using light microscopy and electron microscopy. These data confirm the description above, namely, no scarring inside the cone tip. There are myelinated axons, axo-dendritic synapses, blood vessels, no microglia (that would have indicated gliosis) and no neurons.

students were very interested while more experienced scientists were more skeptical. Having young minds see the potential was extremely encouraging.

The next step was to get FDA approval for human implantation. This was relatively easy to obtain. I say 'relatively' because nowadays you need a whole room full of attorneys to get the FDA's attention! Back in the early 90s I simply sat in the library and made my case to the FDA, sending them all the data I thought they might need. I got back a letter with 21 questions; 13 of the questions where actually answered within the text I had sent. Though that seemed annoying, I realized that I could easily answer the 13 questions. The FDA were pleased and only had eight more questions which I answered almost as easily.

The FDA sent me a short letter giving me permission to implant three patients to make sure that the implantation of the Neurotrophic Electrode would prove to be safe.

The Neurotrophic Electrode is unique because it grows the brain tissue into the Electrode tip thus ensuring longevity of the signal [2][11]. This is unlike all other 'long-term' Electrodes that poke into the brain and lose 85% of signals within three years [3][12]: Not so long-term. This illustration will explain the Neurotrophic Electrode better than my words:

---

[11] *Summary:* The development of a reliable neural interface is essential for lifetime cortical control of prosthetic devices such as robotic arms, paralyzed limbs or speech, and for eventual use in neural augmentation. Standard tine or wire electrodes are not long lasting, surviving a few years with very few remaining useful signals. The Neurotrophic Electrode engages radically different methodology that allows the brain's neuropil to grow into the electrode tip. Six human subjects have been implanted with this electrode, with the longest lasting implant being functional for over 10 years. Eight monkeys and 42 rat implants have also provided valuable experience. Successful anchoring of the electrode tip within the neuropil has resulted in functionally usable single unit recordings over this decade in one human subject. The data presented here include task related cross correlations of neuronal ensembles and reciprocal conditioning of firing rates recorded over the decade. These data demonstrate that stable recordings can be accomplished in humans by *allowing neuropil to grow into the electrode, rather than by inserting the electrode into the neuropil.* This is the first electrode methodology to produce such long-lasting signals that remain functional for over a decade.

[12] *Summary:* This paper admits that new electrodes need to be found rather than the Blackrock array commonly used. These data show that there are 15% single units remaining after 3 years.

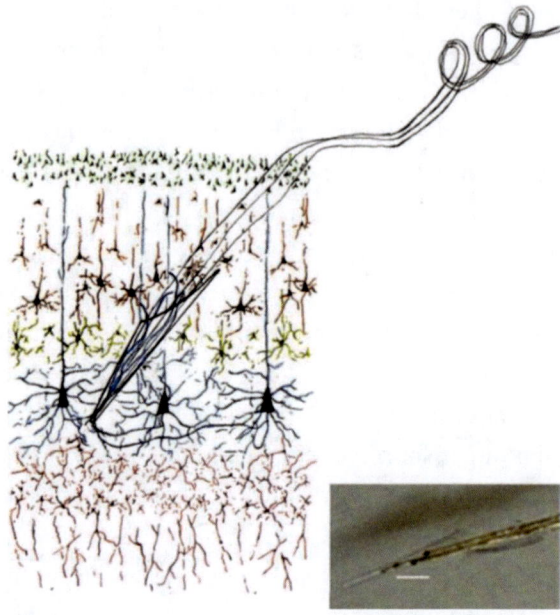

The illustration shows the five layers of motor cortex (from top down). In the deepest area (layer 5) there are large Betz cells that are targeted by the Electrode tip. The tip is a hollow glass cone, coated on the inside with a proprietary mixture of trophic factors to encourage the brain to grow into the tip. Three wires are shown that are coiled for flexibility to allow the Electrode tip to move with the brain. The inset shows a photo of four wires inside the glass tip which is no more than 2 mm in length and a mere 25-50 microns at its deep end. It is several hundred microns at the upper end to allow the wires to enter. The calibration bar marks a distance of 500 μm.

It was in 1996 that Marjorie Hirschberg became the first person to receive the Neurotrophic Electrode. Marjorie demonstrated that she could control the neural signals from her brain, increasing or decreasing the firing activity at our request [4][13], but she did not control the computer. She had ALS and died soon after the implantation from her worsening disease.

In 1998, the second person to participate was Johnny Ray. Johnny remained implanted for four years, and learned to use the computer with the signals from the Electrode. This provided him with slow communication

---

[13] *Summary:* This reports the first person to receive a Neurotrophic Electrode and record from her cortex. She was able to control the firing activity of her neural signals at our request. She could increase and decrease the firing voluntarily. This seminal study lead to further implantations of humans.

such as typing his name, our names and so on [5, 6][14,15]. *He became the world's first cyborg* because he was the first to demonstrate control of a computer 'directly' from his brain. 'Direct' in this context is taken to mean without the usual means of using his arm and fingers to type, mouth to speak and so on. Direct control in this sense does not equate with 'telepathy,' which would imply the transfer of information from one brain to another with no external means of doing so. Instead, what we have done over the past 30+ years is better called 'hard work.'

One thing that disturbed me about the second patient's results was when we realized that he had some muscle activity in his neck and face. I reasoned that unless somebody was completely 'locked-in,' it would not be justified to implant them just to control the computer because, after all, the muscle activity could be used to control the computer (without the risk of brain surgery and the presence of foreign material within the skull). So we also developed an alternate system to use residual muscle activity to control the computer. But that is a story for another day. What I realized is that the implantation we performed would no longer be ethical just to spell on the computer. Having thought about it for quite some time I came to the conclusion that it would be justifiable, however, to implant the brain of a human to restore fine finger movements or to restore speech because these activities require high resolution signals that are only found from individual neurons in the cortex. The Neurotrophic Electrode can offer that opportunity despite being a fully locked-in subject.

---

[14] *Summary:* Person JR was the first to control a computer allowing him to spell his name and our names, as well as outputting the words via the computer speaker. He was implanted in his hand motor cortex and had auditory feedback of the firing of single units and visual feedback of the cursor. These data demonstrate learning of the tasks and thus improvements in his speed of communication. They demonstrate improved scoring within a few trials and breakdown of the learning when fatigued. Target accuracy improved when moving the cursor either with a few single units or just one.

[15] *Summary:* These data were also acquired from person JR and relate to characteristics of the data. He was implanted in the hand area of motor cortex. Initially, he was thinking of moving his hand to activate the neural signal firings. Later, when we asked what he was thinking, he spelled out: "nothing." The next day we asked him again, and he spelled out "moving the cursor." This was the first documented example of "cursor related cortex," that is, the cursor being incorporated into his body image.

We next implanted a person, Tim Tinius, with mitochondrial myopathy which is a muscle disease that leaves someone paralyzed, able to think but not speak. The literature at the time indicated that it was a disease of muscle *only*, but we were shocked to find it affected the brain also. So that was a blank test. Then, finally, we implanted David Jayne, the patient with ALS, in the hand area of his brain and indeed showed that the neural signals were related to his muscle activity. However, the implanted electrode and electronics, disappointingly, had to be removed soon after implantation due to the fact that the incision was not closing fully. As Florence Nightingale and Thomas Sydenham said, first do no harm!

So let's talk specifically about Erik, whose injury provided us with both a unique opportunity and a very real challenge.

Chapter 11

ERIK'S INJURY

In brief, the car flipped over three times into a ditch. Erik was the passenger. The driver was unhurt. No drugs or alcohol were involved. Erik was transported into the emergency room of Gwinnett Medical Center. After surgery to repair his fractures and remove his bleeding spleen, he appeared to be unconscious. However, he was seen to blink. Tests of his blood vessels showed an interruption of his basilar artery, a vessel critical to feeding the brainstem. It shut off. He had a brainstem stroke. He was locked-in. His parents were devastated.

He spent weeks in intensive care, followed by several months in the Shepperd Rehabilitation Center. It was there that his parents learned how to care for him at home: Managing the ventilator, suctioning his lungs, supplying the stomach feeding tube with liquid nutrition, turning him in bed frequently to avoid the formation of bedsores, all that was their heroic lot for the next 18 years. Ten years after the electrode implantation, his blood pressure became very unstable, perhaps by spreading of his stroke to involve autonomic systems or their descending pathways in the brainstem so that his blood pressure became highly unstable. This eventually prevented him from even raising his head without passing out, preventing further recording. Thus, recording ended in 2014. Erik died in the fall of 2017. His recordings 'moved the needle' for locked-in people. Yes, he produced words, but no, he could not speak spontaneously. However, he showed the way forward.

Chapter 12

MEETING DR. KENNEDY

As mentioned above, Erik's dad Eddie Ramsey, called me. We got together and I explained the pros and cons of the experiment to him, his wife and to Erik. I mentioned that we had implanted four people since 1996, demonstrating how the brain signals could provide communication. I told them that we were more ambitious and wanted to restore speech. Of course, I explained to them that this might not work, or that the success might only be partial. I also told them about myself. I explained how I had received an MD degree from the National University in Ireland in 1976, a surgical degree from the Royal College of Surgeons in Ireland in 1978, had worked in neurosurgery for a few years and then went into research at the University of Western Ontario, Canada, had received a PhD from Northwestern University in Chicago Illinois in 1983 and began work on the Neurotrophic Electrode in 1986 by implanting rat brains. These initial implants demonstrated clearly that the brain tissue could grow into the tip of the Electrode and remain there for the lifetime of the rat (16 months). I explained how the Electrode is a piece of a glass capillary measuring 2 mm in length, 300 microns at the upper end and as little as 25 to 50 microns at the deep end [1][16]. A few Teflon insulated 2 mil gold wires are glued inside by entering the wide upper end and using methyl methacrylate glue (routinely

---

[16] See reference summary on page 91.

used by neurosurgeons). I explained to them how the histological data showed the brain sending tendrils of neurons (neurites) into the glass cone, and that we had not seen scarring (gliosis) that would impede the recording of signals over time [7][17]. The secret to getting the ingrowth: Using trophic factors to entice the brain to grow into the glass tip. Another big bonus: Long-term recording. All Neurotrophic Electrodes continued recording until the person died or the implant had to be removed. In Erik it lasted a decade up to his death [2][18]. Other types of Electrodes poke into the brain and their recordings do not endure due to a) scarring which separates the recording tip from the neurons, and b) micromovements of the tip relative to the neurons so that the neural signals wax and wane.

I also explained to Erik and his parents that the signals are extracted from the brain using an amplifier attached to the electrode wires. This is powered by a power induction coil which is applied to the scalp to turn on the system and continuously power the device. This power also drives a transmitter unit that broadcasts the neural signals using FM across the scalp. Thus no wires exit the scalp thereby reducing the possibility of introducing infection. Problems? Yes, of course. Each implanted recording device is a single channel and no more than three could be implanted, thus reducing the number of signals that could be recorded. However, each pair of wires could record 15 to 20 single units so we could get a reasonable number of signals that might be adequate to produce speech. Furthermore, there is a delay of three to four months while the neurites are growing in and are useful. However, a few months in the lifetime of a locked-in person waiting for the electrode to become active is hardly a disadvantage. On the plus side, we learned from the rat studies that the neurons that sent in the neurites are spread out for a millimeter or more around the tip so that we record from a wide area of the brain, or at least wide enough to harvest adequate signals for speech. Not only that, but neurites grow in the top end of the Neurotrophic Electrode have different characteristics from those that grow in the lower end so they can be easily distinguished.

---

[17] See reference summary on page 90.
[18] See reference summary on page 91.

So Erik's dad and mom discussed the pros and cons with Erik. They all agreed to go ahead. They signed the Human Investigation Committee's paperwork on Erik's behalf and with his agreement.

Chapter 13

THE IMPLANT SURGERY

On December 22nd 2004, Erik was implanted with an Neurotrophic Electrode into his motor cortex near his speech area. Two electronic wireless devices were attached and recordings began a few months later after the brain elements had grown into the electrode.

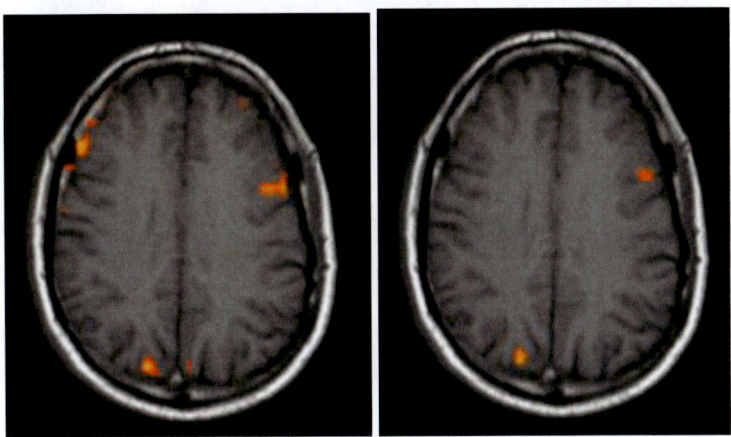

The target area for implantation was determined by functional Magnetic Resonance Imaging (MRI). A regular MRI demonstrates the anatomic structure of the brain, whereas a functional MRI indicates where a function is taking place. In Erik's case, since he was mute, we had him look at pictures of dogs, cats, alligators and so on. His task was to say in his head "This is a dog, this a cat," etc. That activity showed up on the functional MRI as shown below. An example is shown here for audible speech on the left panel and silent speech on the right (not Erik's). That yellow/red area became our target. This was not necessarily in the most lateral part of the motor cortex which is where we now know the speech articulators are controlled. We simply went with the functional MRI result. Note the smaller area for silent speech. This area is on the right side of the MRI (that is the left side of the brain). The 'hot' spot at the back is in the occipital or *visual* cortex, that lights up due to looking at the picture.

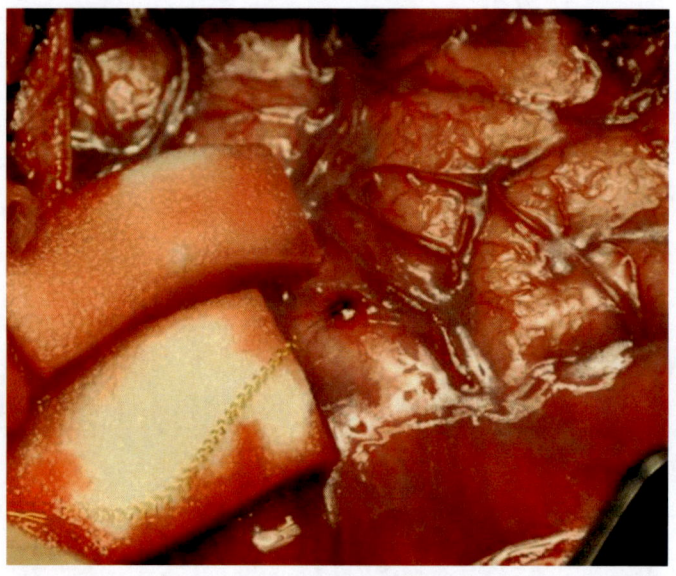

After induction of anesthesia, Erik's head was shaved and cleaned with an antiseptic solution. His scalp was opened and a portion of his skull removed over the target. This craniotomy allowed us to peer onto his brain surface (cortex) and match the functional MRI findings with his actual cortex, thereby determining the target for implantation. A small incision was made into the cortex and the electrode tip was gently inserted into the cortex, to a depth of 6 mm at an angle of 45 degrees. The center of the figure shows the opening in the cortex where the electrode enters and the coiled electrode wire is seen lower left. This photograph is from a different case.

The Implant Surgery

After the electrodes were in place, the wireless electronics were connected. An x-ray from a different case is shown here to illustrate the position of the electronics and the electrode wires (in this case three sets of wireless electronics). The electrode wires are seen near the center of the Xray. These wires lead to connectors and then to the amplifers and FM transmitters. The device is powered by power induction with the receiving coils above (they look as if they are floating. They are not!). The power induction works like an electric toothbrush that is placed in its inductive holder. During use, an external coil is placed outside the scalp over the inner induction coil to send power to the amplifier and transmitter. Then an FM receiving coil is placed over the FM transmitter to receive the data. The recordings began several months after the surgery to allow time for the brain tissue to grow in. The results of these recordings are described in the following chapters.

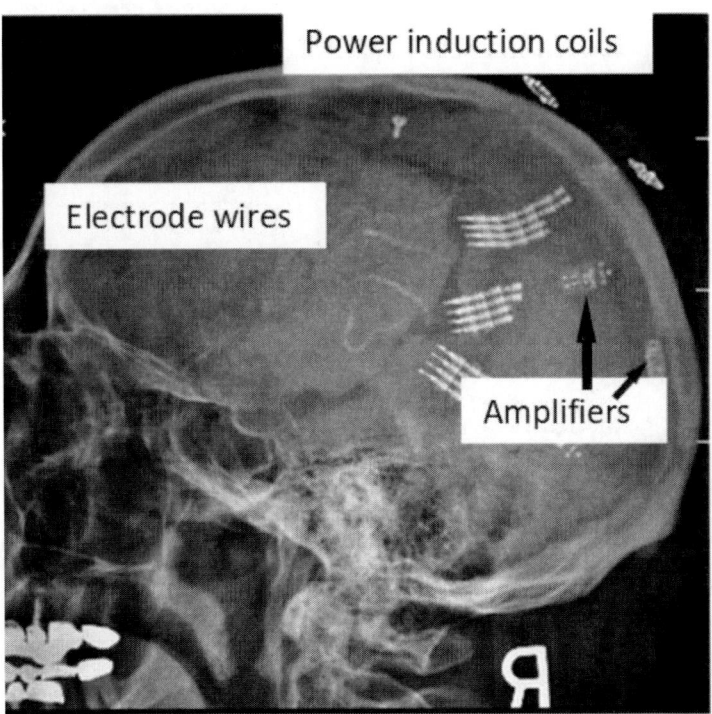

Chapter 14

RECORDING FROM ERIK

Three days a week for many years, Erik sat in his wheel chair and was brought by his Dad to the laboratory. To set up the recording, we first placed the coils on Erik's head as shown in the picture here:

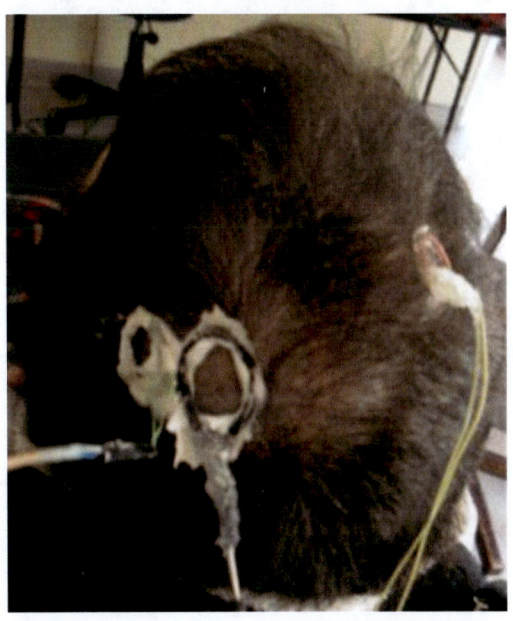

This view of Erik's head is from behind and shows the power induction coil on the right and the two FM receiving coils on the left. The white paste is water soluble EEG glue that holds the coil firmly in place and is easily wiped off with water after the recording session is finished. The power induction coil is over the inner power cords that you can see in the x-ray. There are two FM receiving coils on the left that take the FM carrier signals to receivers that will remove the neural signals from the FM carriers. These signals are continuous and they are archived for later retrieval. The continuous signal also goes to a computer where signals from individual neurites are detected. Here is an example of that process.

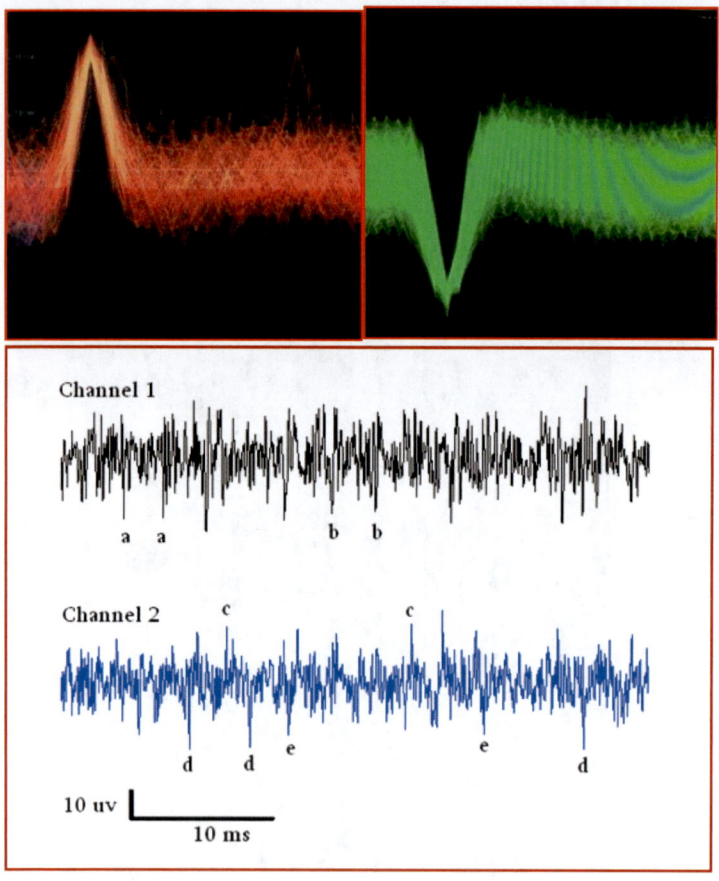

There are two coils because there are two amplifiers and hence two channels of continuous data (left). You can see the similar spikes of single units labelled 'a,' 'b,' 'c,' etc. These are separated from the continuous signal by a software program [9]. This produces single 'units' as shown here.

You will notice that some units are upgoing and some down going, as shown in both the continuous data stream and in the single units. It is these single units that are the keys to decoding the data.

Chapter 15

USING SINGLE UNITS TO SAY "DA, DA"

One of the first attempts was to link single units to words. First a little history: Eb Fetz and colleagues had published way back in 1973 that monkeys could control the activity of single nerve cells for a juice reward [8][19]. In fact, the monkeys could control two nerve cells at the same time by making the firing of one unit increase while the other decreased. We figured that Erik could do this too.

So, using software, we built wavefiles that when activated would output words such as "DA" or "MA" and several others through the computer speakers so Erik would get the reward of hearing himself speak. We linked those wavefiles to the activity of single nerve cells recorded from Erik's brain so that when these 'units' fired, the wavefiles were triggered to produce the words.

The computer first said the words twice and Erik had to repeat them. He could do it as you can see in this video (ErikSingleUnitsWords.url). It can

---

[19] These data demonstrated that monkeys could modulate firing rates of single units recorded from motor cortex. The monkeys visualized a needle on a rate meter while the researchers recorded single units from the motor cortex. It was possible to record more than one unit, so in that case, the monkeys were rewarded with fruit juice to increase the rate of one unit while at the same time decreasing the rate of the other unit. This was the first demonstration that differential conditioning of single units was possible.

be a little puzzling at first to know which is the computer and which is Erik 'speaking,' so here is a key.

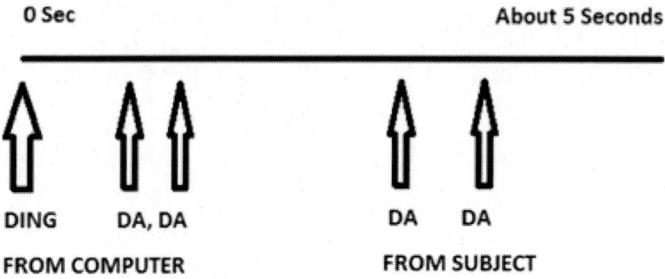

When you go to the *.url* on www.neuralsignlas.com web site you will see this picture first. Click on it to listen to Erik 'saying' Da, Da.

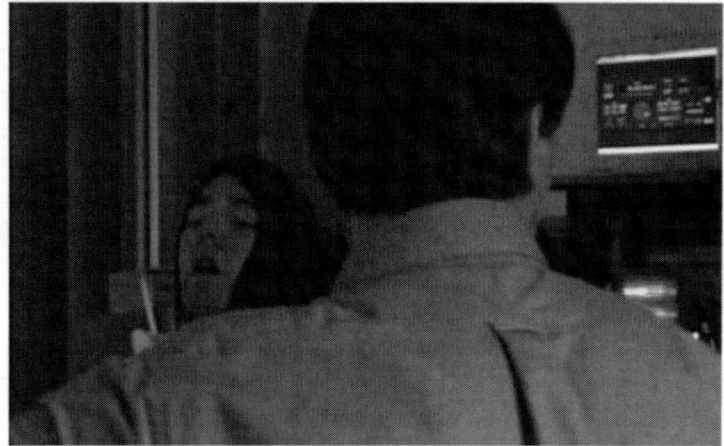

Erik told us that he loved doing this test. He was thrilled to hear himself 'speak.' But there was a problem: It ought to be theoretically possible to link 100 useful words to 100 single units and for Erik to control them all. But that is not how the brain works. It works in *patterns* of single units firing.

So we changed our approach and set out to detect the patterns.

Chapter 16

DECODING 22 TO 24 OF 39 PHONES

Phones are the building blocks of words. Say 'aaah,' say 'eeeh,' say 'mmm,' these are all phones. For example, the spoken word Dad consists of three phones, 'dah,' 'ah,' and 'dah.' All in all, there are 39 phones in the English language. By decoding the ensemble of brain activity, 22-24 phones were detected in Erik by decoding the *patterns* of single unit firings.

The way we found out about this was to examine the firing of single units while he said 'Dad' in his head. We had him repeat the word 10 times while we recorded the single units. Remember that he was saying it in his head so we had no direct indication that he was saying it. We asked him afterwards if he was speaking in his head. He turned his eyes up for 'yes' and down for 'no,' and he usually turned his eyes up. Note that we were not asking him to imagine the phones, we wanted him to actually say them as if he could speak. This brings up a huge problem for this work: how can we verify that he is, in fact, speaking in his head and when exactly does he start speaking? For the starting point, we could not simply speak the phone to him while he spoke in his head because the single unit responses could be just auditory input due to us speaking the phones. To avoid this confound, we played the phones three times and then asked him to say them silently in his head. We had to trust that he was being truthful, that he was not fatigued and so on. But that is one major reasons why I decided later that I should consider implanting myself so I could speak out loud and then speak silently in my head. More on that later beginning in chapter 19.

So to decode the phones we examined the patterns of firing of the single units. The patterns were sufficiently different, allowing us to differentiate 22-24 phones from the total of 39 with some accuracy as shown in this figure.

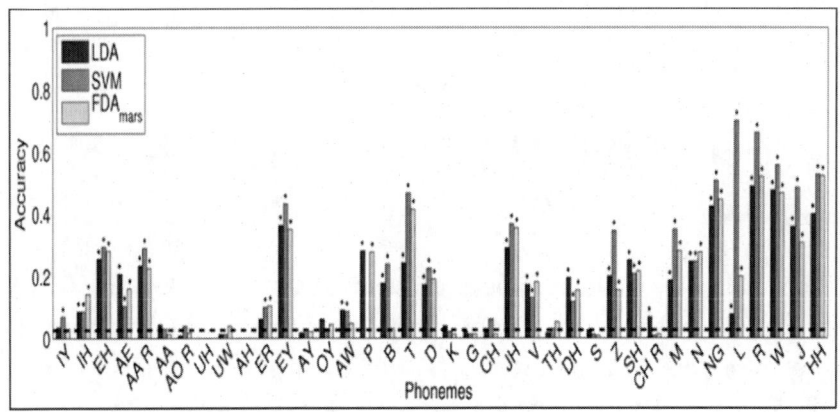

On the X-axis, the vowel phones are the 15 on the left, and the consonants are on the right. The accuracy is shown on the Y-axis with 1 being strongest possible certainty of identification. The consonants on the right are clearly more strongly identified than the vowels though none reach a level of 1. Three computer programs LDA, SVM and FDA (in box top left) were used and their results mostly agree [10], with the SVM producing the highest accuracy. The dashed line is the chance level, so 24 phones are detected above this line. Applying the criterion that all three decoding paradigms had to be significantly above chance (the dashed line in the figure), leaves us with 22 of 39 decoded.

Chapter 17

MOVING FROM VOWEL TO VOWEL

After identifying the phones, we sought to use them to create speech. A team led by Professor Frank Guenther and Jon Brumberg, a Boston University doctoral candidate worked with us. Jon ran the experiments from Boston using a microphone and speaker, and by controlling our computers from his Boston lab. It was almost as if Jon was in the room with us!

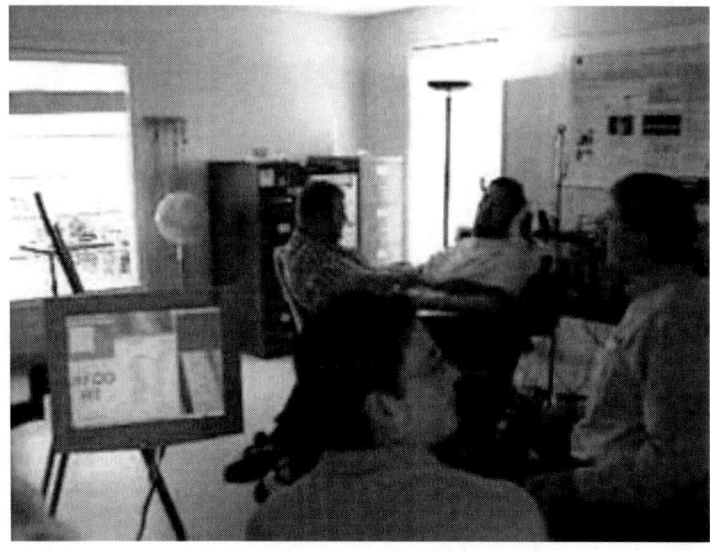

He *was* in the room with us at the beginning of the experiments as you can see from the photos! In the wheelchair you can see Erik with his Dad in front of him. I can be seen at right. Jon is closest. So go to the *.url* (www.neuralsignals.com) and see what we found. Before you go there, let me explain a few things.

This is a 2D format frequency plane:

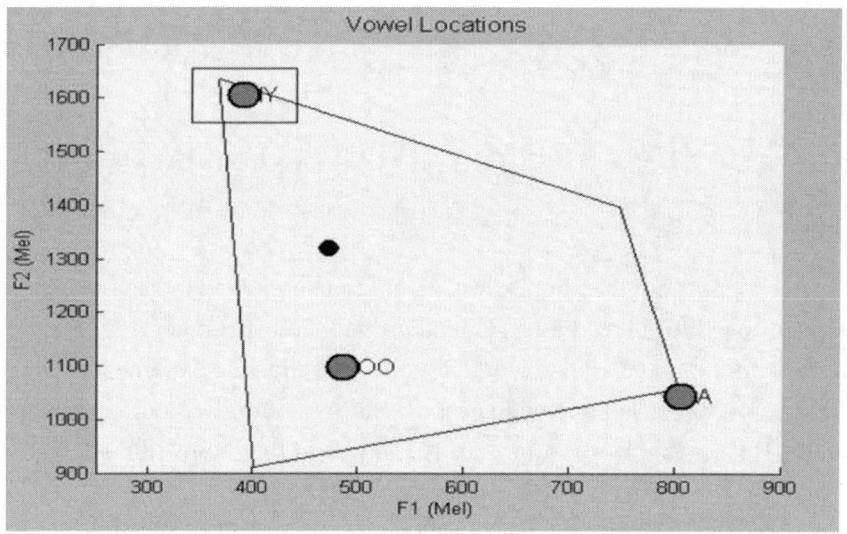

This is the screen that Erik looked at during the study. Note that the X-axis frequencies go from low to high left to right, and the Y-axis frequencies do the same thing from below to above but at higher frequencies than on the X-axis.

If the cursor (represented by a dark brown dot) is moved to a high area it sounds like an 'eeeeh' and low down is sounds like an 'uuuuh' and down to the right it sounds like 'aaaah.'

Moving the cursor around the 2D formant plane produces vowel sounds, in fact all vowel sounds in the English language. Erik's task would be to move the cursor and produce the sounds. In case you think we invented this, let's back up and look at history.

Moving from Vowel to Vowel

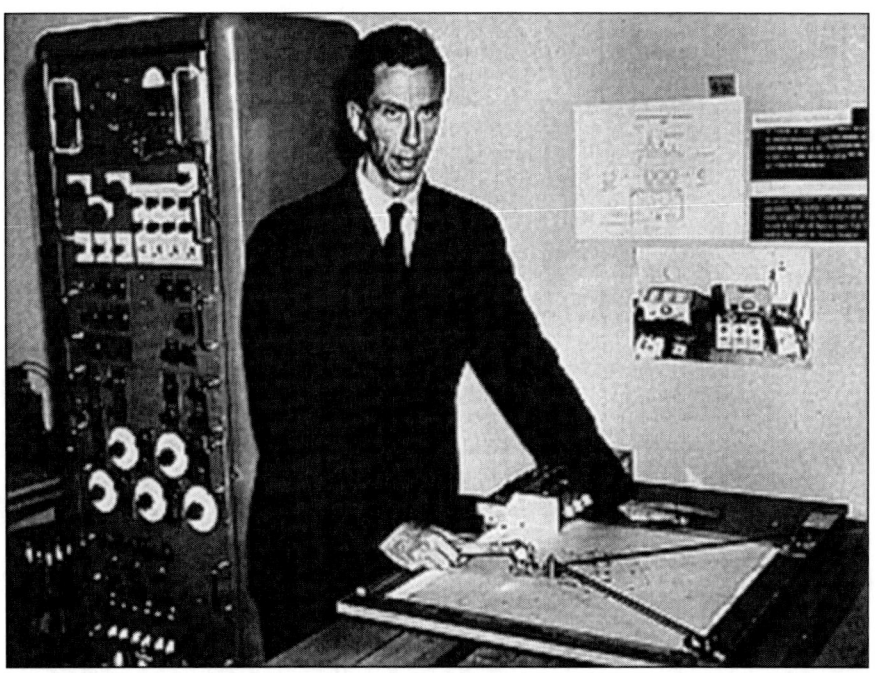

This is a 1953 photo of Gunner Fant, the inventor of the *Orator Verbis Electris*. He developed the electronics that can be seen in the background (it was ahead of its time then!) and he is holding a handle on the board in front of him.

The board is actually our friend: the 2D formant frequency plane! When he moved it around he could produce vowels, but not only vowels, soft consonants as well. He was able to say "How are you? I love you." He produced the soft consonants such as 'L' by swiftly moving the handle against the side of the board.

Back to Erik and Jon: With this background you should be able to listen to what happens when Erik moves the cursor around on the 2D formant frequency plane. How did he do it? Jon wrote the software to translate the firing *patterns* of single units into movements of the cursor across the 2D plane. Erik could produce the patterns and learnt to do it well as you can see from these plots.

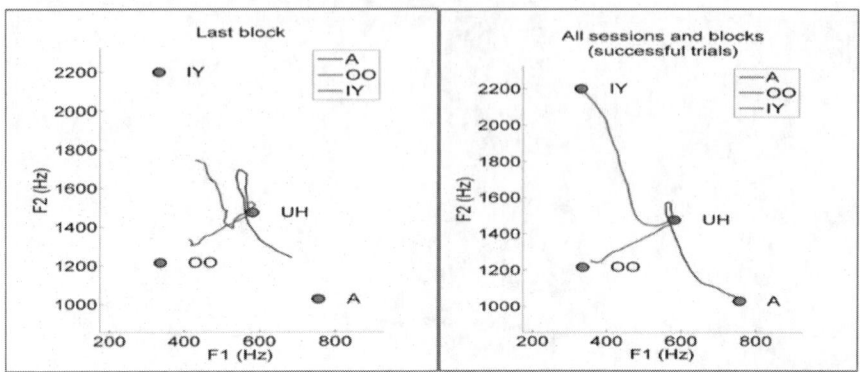

On the left, the squiggly lines show his initial attempts to move around the plane, but after many weeks of training he did very well (right panel).

After you look at the .url ( ) I will explain the problem with this approach.

Back to the problem with this approach. Let me explain with a simple plot. This is the time it took to achieve the vowel target so you can clearly see that taking about 4 seconds will not produce anywhere near normal speech.

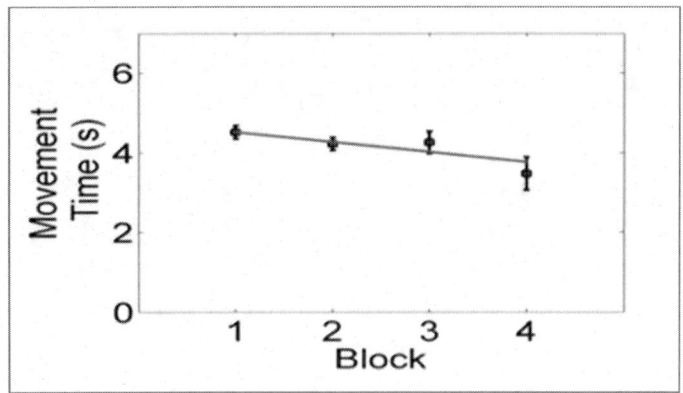

If we want to generate speech of normal speed, we obviously have to think of another way to do this. We found a way but did not achieve it with Erik. Let us first look at some of the other problems such as the effect of emotion on firing rates.

Chapter 18

THE EFFECTS OF EMOTION ON FIRING RATES

We had noticed in Erik and previously implanted people that the firing rates were very variable. We first realized this in 1998 with our subject Johnny Ray (JR). JR, like Erik, had a brainstem stroke and was paralyzed and mute except for some face movements. When we were setting up the recording system he watched us intently and single units fired actively. However, as soon as we turned to him to start working, the firing stopped. At first we thought the units were lost. But the firing picked up again after he got to work attempting to control the cursor. We determined to explore this further.

We had the opportunity with Erik. On day 1412 after implantation, Erik was performing a task for several minutes as illustrated in the figure, red panel. Channel 1 data are above and channel 2 data below in the figure where each row represents the firing rate of recorded units, the higher the bars, the faster the rate. He then took a break as illustrated in the green panel, when he nodded off to sleep. Activity on all channels quietened down somewhat during sleep. Eight minutes later we turned on music to wake him up (blue panel): Channel 2 became active again, but not channel 1. After a break, we next turned the room light on for over a minute and then off (brown area indicates 'on' and dark green area indicates 'off'). There was little or no change in firing rates on both channels. The room lights were still on, as were colored lights from the electronics behind him. We then plunged the room into almost total darkness as shown in the black area labeled 'D' by turning off the projector, the overhead and the backlights. Some colored light remained from the computer displays behind the subject. This had a marked increase in firing rates of channel 1 units, but had little effect on the firing rates of units on channel 2. When the room lights were turned back on (yellow area) there was only a small effect on the firing rates in either channel mainly affecting the slower firing units. When his Dad entered the room however, there was a further dramatic generalized increase in channel 1 firings but no effect on channel 2 firings.

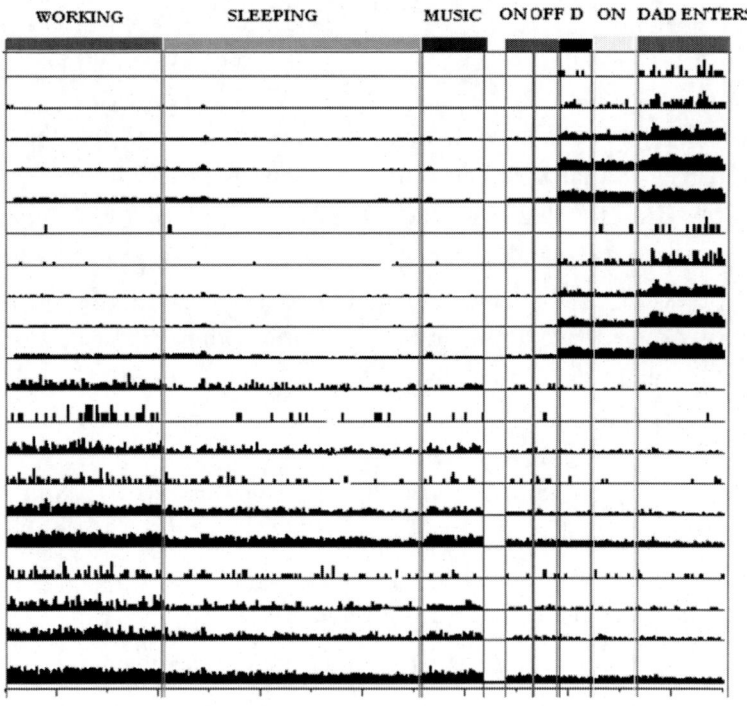

100 SECS

We interpreted these results as follows: As expected with working, units were active that then quietened down when he fell asleep. Waking him with music had little effect on firing. Turning lights on or off had no effect. However, plunging the room into darkness produced a dramatic increase in firing because as he told us he was *afraid of the dark*. So emotion drove the increase. When his dad came *into the room* there was a dramatic increase in firing. The emotion of seeing his dad produced increases in firing. Further control studies confirmed these results. This study was published as a case report [11][20].

The importance of these results is that variable firing is something we had to learn to accommodate. Stabilizing the subject's change in emotion (such as seeing his Dad) before and during recording was always essential.

---

[20] This paper describes modulations in firing rates during changes in emotion. When Erik's dad comes into the room, very quiet firings suddenly light up. This is described in the text.

Chapter 19

MUSIC RELATES TO FIRING RATES

A fun and surprising part of our work with Erik had to do with music.

Erik loved music! His favorite group was Slipknot. He used to go to concerts with his friends and have lots of fun. He liked to listen to music while we fussed around the lab getting everything ready. So we continued to have him listen to music while we recorded his neural signals. What we found relates to music and learning.

In the figure below you can see examples of slow firing, medium firing, fast firing and fastest firing nerve cells recorded on days 1546, 1549, 1553 and 1556 after implantation. The firing rates are shown in the Y axis. The paradigm was to have Erik first listen to the 523 Hz tone (high 'C') for 10 seconds, followed by a 10 second quiet period, that was followed by him trying to hum the tone in his head for 10 seconds, all repeated 10 times. So each wavy line has these three points showing the firing rates during these three 10 second periods. On days 1546 and 1549, he received no feedback of the tone when he tried to hum it in his head. On day 1553, he received a feedback of the tone when he hummed it. Notice how the firing rates go from being disorganized the first two days to somewhat organized when he received the feedback. When he received feedback that became louder and louder as the firing rate increased on day 1556, the firing became highly organized. This is shown on the panel on the right. This was a big surprise!

Also, when the tone was changed to 262 Hz (middle 'C') the pattern changed suggesting that the pattern was specific for specific tones. This is very obvious for single units labelled CH2-17 and ch2-9. This was fascinating to us because it was not the auditory cortex but the speech motor cortex.

Notice also that the pattern of organization of the firing rates was gradually acquired over the 10 repetitions. This is a classic learning pattern. So Erik could learn to fire his neurons. That is important in developing prostheses because it suggests that a neuron related to one action can be trained to drive a different action.

But there is more to this story. See next chapter.

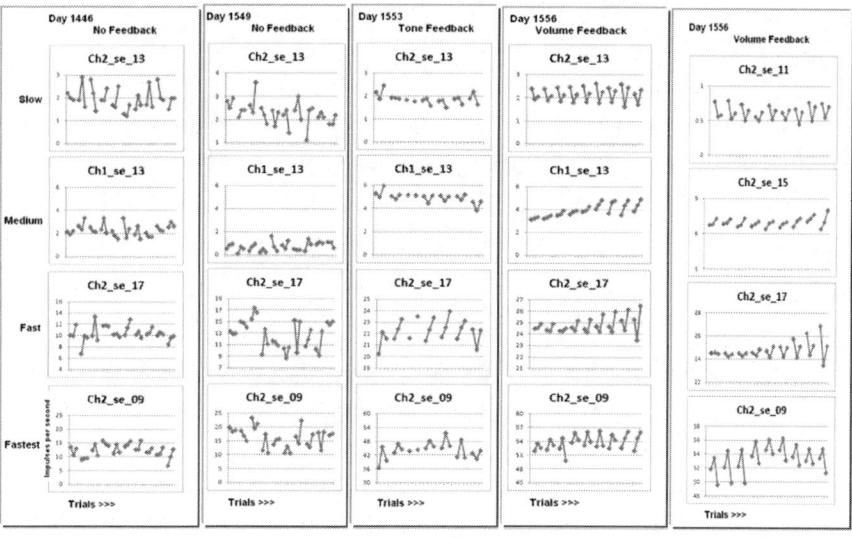

Chapter 20

CONDITIONING SINGLE UNITS NINE YEARS AFTER IMPLANTATION

A big question in this study was whether or not the Neurotrophic Electrode would survive for several years. It did. The evidence is in this chapter. Erik's electronics broke down and were replaced eight years after implantation. Erik agreed to be recorded again at year nine. By year ten his stroke had spread to the blood pressure control area in his brain stem and he would pass out every time he lifted his head.

So we are lucky to be able to record at years nine and ten.

We performed several conditioning studies to demonstrate that the single units were still useful and not just noise in the system. Because he had done well with the tone study related above, we repeated this as follows. Several years previously he had responded to a guitar note with high firing in unit number ch2-se-17. This is unit 18 in the figure below. These units were all recorded on day 3135 after implantation and rates were normalized by taking the ratio of task-related firings (averaged over 10 seconds) *after* the 'go' signal (listening to the guitar note) and compared them with 10 second averages *before* the 'go' signal. The ratio does not increase for most units on this day 3135 except for ch2-se-17 (now #18). However, four days later (day 3139), the same paradigm suggested that unit SE2_se_17 (the previously conditioned unit, now #18) did dramatically increase its ratio on the second set (purple bar) and maintained this increase on the third set (yellow bar). Most other units also increased their ratios, at least by the third set, to some degree, but ch2-se-17 (#18) was the standout champion in response to that tone.

This example [21] and several others suggested to us that the single units can *endure* and can be *conditioned*. That is a really important finding. Also of great interest is that the unit being conditioned in year nine was also responsive to the same guitar note several years before!

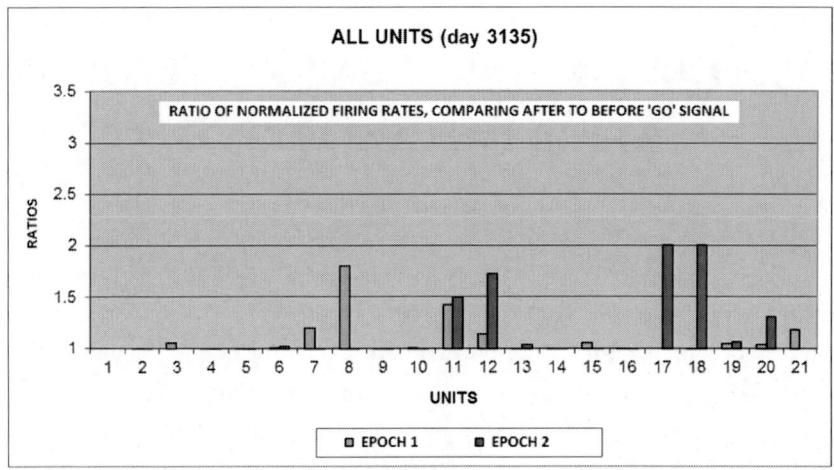

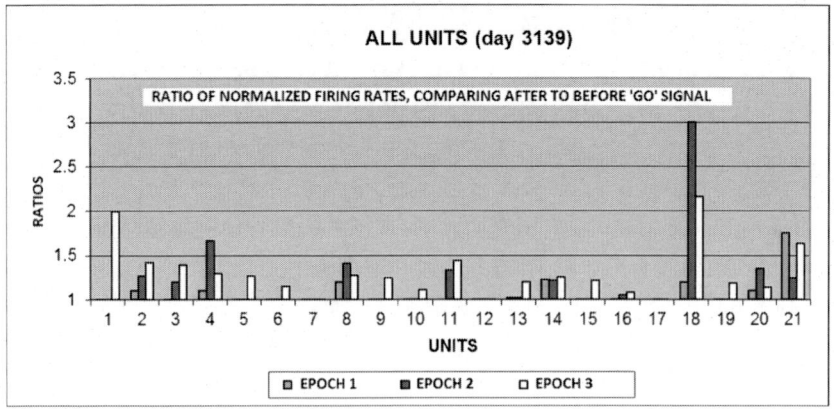

Chapter 21

LIMITATIONS OF ERIK'S RECORDINGS

Sadly, we did not get Erik to speak. We learned a lot and feel confident we can achieve our goal thanks to his courageous efforts and tireless work in the laboratory.

There were several limitations to the recordings. First there were never enough single units. A few dozen in Erik was good but a few hundred would have been better. The limitation was due to the limited number of amplifiers and transmitters that could be placed under the scalp. We now know that four electrodes with two pairs of wires in each would be sufficient if placed in the approximately one inch diameter cortex where the neural controllers of the articulators reside. Each electrode records from about a 2 mm diameter around the deep tip of the electrode. Of importance, the electrodes, when spaced 6 mm apart, would sample from almost the whole speech motor cortex. Each electrode pair records about 15 to 20 single units. With four electrodes, each with 2 pairs of wires, that is 8 pairs times 20 single units would give us 160 units. That should be plenty.

Another limitation was that we could not know when Erik was about to start 'speaking.' One way around that problem would be to implant the electrodes in an ALS patient who was still speaking and then follow the signals as speech was invariably lost. However, it would be obviously highly unethical to carry out a speech prosthesis experiment in a vulnerable ALS patient still able to speak, risking the catastrophic outcome that he/she might lose speech due to the implantation procedure. The only way to carry out this experiment was to implant a person who could speak audibly and silently, and, importantly, would be willing to risk losing essential neurological function as the result of this study: myself.

Chapter 22

PHIL'S IMPLANTATION SURGERY

So, on June 21st 2014 I went to Belize under the care of Dr. Cervantes, a neurosurgeon. He was trained in Mexico City and from previous observations at surgery I could see that he was an excellent neurosurgeon. I trusted him to carry out a Neurotrophic Electrode implantation procedure on my brain. I also knew all the possible things that could go wrong after surgery. And many did go wrong. I had performed this surgery on 42 rat brains, 8 monkeys (with Dr. Bakay a neurosurgeon) and had attended all human implantations of course, so I had figured out the complications. One complication would be permanent loss of speech, so I had prepared computer programs to allow me to speak slowly using finger tapping of icons and words if that happened.

The plan was to implant four Neurotrophic Electrodes 6 mm apart within the motor speech cortex. This area lies just above the Sylvian fissure that demarcates the lowest part of the motor cortex from the temporal cortex. This fissure can be found by placing your finger tip one inch above the spot where your ear meets your scalp. The figure of my brain implantation is above in chapter 3 where Erik's surgery is described. I had essentially the same procedure as Erik, with the exception that four electrodes with four wires in each were implanted. I had expected to externalize the connectors so I built big connectors as can be seen in the X ray in chapter 3. Alas, the neurosurgeons would not allow me to externalize the electrode connectors, even though it is routinely done by other researchers. I wanted to externalize the electrodes so I could record from them all and have many units. So, instead, in October 2014 three electronic single channel wireless devices were placed under the scalp as can be seen in the X ray in chapter 3. This allowed me to record from only three of the electrodes and usually only one at a time.

Immediately after the 12-hour surgery in June 2014, I felt fine. I was speaking and waking up normally with very little pain in the incision. The next day however, I lost my speech. Not only that, I could not write. I knew what I wanted to say and write, but I could not! My comprehension was intact, but writing and speaking were impossible. I had some brain swelling which is understandable considering four electrodes were tightly placed in a small area. A CT scan showed the swelling. I was also limping on my right side. In addition, I developed focal seizures in my right jaw which required medication. I received medications to reduce the swelling. Five days later, my speech began to recover and my weakness improved. The weakness was due to the swelling of surrounding motor cortex. It took another three months for the speech to recover fully. I had no more focal seizures after a few days and was able to stop the medications 6 months later, without recurrence of seizures.

The next step, mentioned above, took place in October 2014, when three wireless electronic devices were placed under my scalp and attached to some of the electrode pairs as can be seen in the X ray in chapter 3. There was not enough room to place more than three. Shortly after that, I began to record neural signals in the laboratory. I was able to record a total of 65 single units, 21, 21 and 23 in electrodes 1, 2 and 3 respectively.

Chapter 23

SENSORY AND MOTOR RELATIONSHIPS

The first thing I did was to decide if the electrode was in the speech motor cortex. It was. But I got a surprise!

How is this done? Simply by looking at the firing rates after making movements of the lips, tongue, jaw and larynx. The result is shown here:

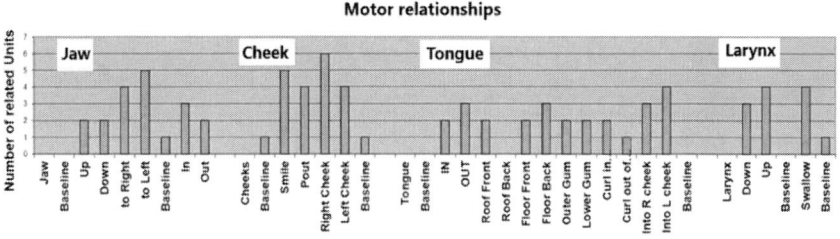

As an example, jaw movements to right or to left caused as many as 4 or 5 single units to fire. The electrical activity (EMG) from the jaw muscles cannot interfere since the recording is from inside the glass cone only, and not attached to a ground which could have picked up muscle activity. Baseline is simply not moving anything. With cheek movements, a smile or right and left cheek movements caused 5 or 6 single units to fire. And so on for the tongue and larynx.

But here comes the surprise: Single units also fired to light touch and pin prick. Wait! This was supposed to be a motor area only? Yes, but even motor areas have sensory inputs and hence sensory responses. Afterall, there has to be a connection between sensory and motor. See the data here:

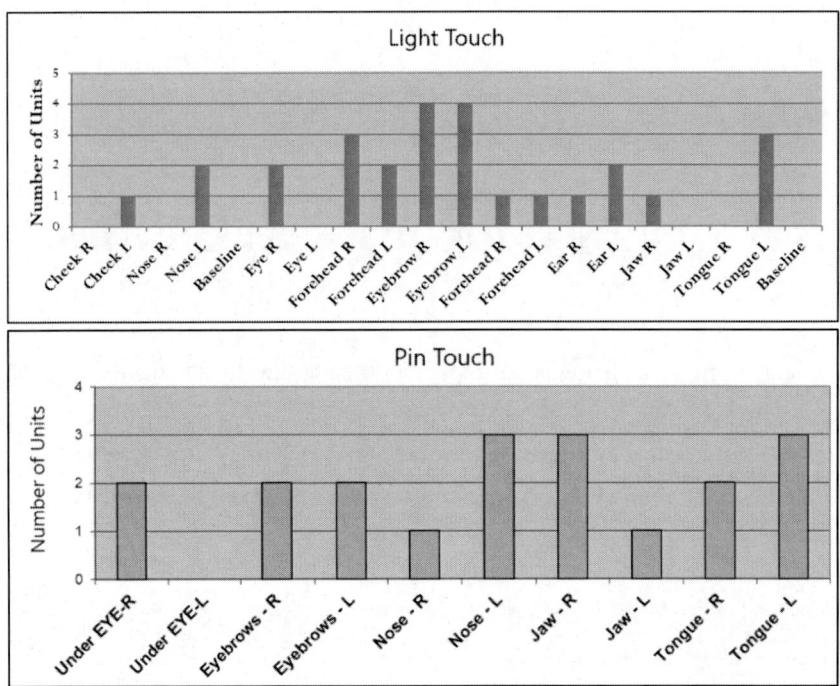

Look carefully at the labels on the figure. Can you see something odd? The eyes, eyebrows, forehead and even the ear provoked some single unit firings. They are far away from the mouth. Right? Wrong: When we speak we use expressions and move our facial muscles: Our whole face becomes involved. So of course there are sensory and motor responses to the whole face.

Once I knew that the electrodes were implanted in the correct area and had these data, I went ahead to examine components of speech such as phones, words and phrases.

Chapter 24

DECODING MOST PHONES

Recall that phones are the building blocks of language. For example, say 'eh,' 'uh' 'oh' and so on. These can be built into words such as 'bed,' 'put' and 'hold.' So to detect phones is the first step in decoding language. There are 39 phones in the English language.

There were three active electrodes in my brain, the third being the closest to my ear. The electrode wires are shown on the X ray in chapter 3. In one simple experiment, I said the phones 10 times and looked for increases in firing of the single units. The results are shown in the figures below for the three electrodes. The vowels are on the left side of the X axis and the consonants are on the right side. The number of single units that responded to phones are shown on the Y axis. As you can see, electrode 1 had more single unit responses to vowels, whereas electrode 2 had somewhat more single unit responses to consonants. electrode 3 was the most responsive to both vowels and consonants. From the work of Chang et al. [17, 18] we know there is a layout, with the vowels more medial and consonants more lateral (towards the ear). So these data approximately agree with their data. The gaps in the histogram display are units that did not respond. Some phones had very few single unit responses.

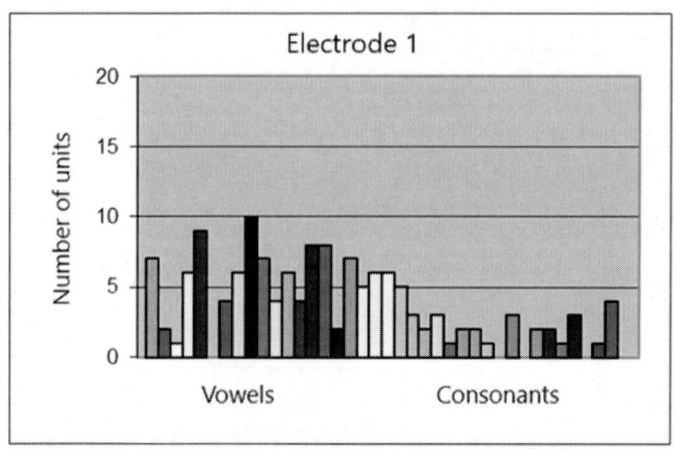
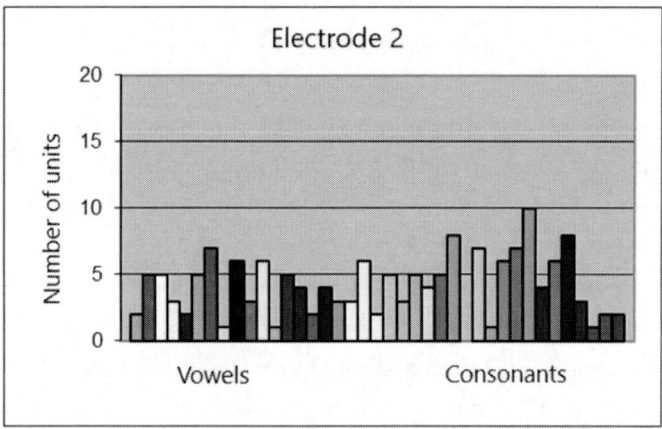
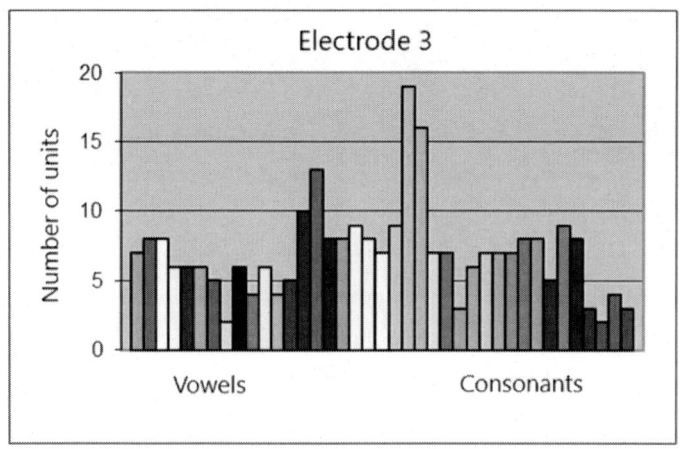

Overall, most phones were detected using only 65 single units. With a larger number of single units it is likely that all phones would be detected, but that is for another day!

Chapter 25

DECODING AUDIBLE AND SILENT SPEECH

So, once we knew that most phones would respond to single unit firings, we determined to see if audible and silent phrases could be decoded [22]. Decoding silent phrases is of course the ultimate aim, which is to assist locked-in folks to speak at near conversational rates. I spoke phrases 10 times out loud and then spoke them again 10 times *silently*. I placed a marker on the data to determine the onset of audible and silent speech. To decode those phrases, I at first used the single units on their own. This was helpful but not good enough. So, we looked at the patterns of single unit bursts as shown here.

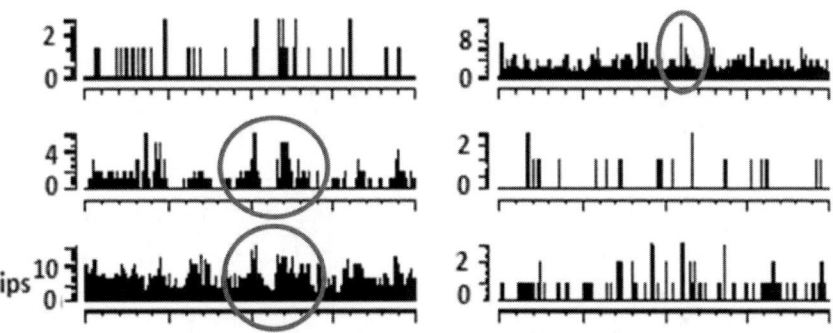

Examples of single unit bursts

It is easy to see a burst and then a silent period and then another burst on the left side of the figure (circled in red). On the right there is simply a burst (circled in red). The other three examples have no clear bursts. 'ips' means impulses per second. The time scale is not relevant because this is just an example to demonstrate the bursts.

The next step was to classify the bursts as numbers as shown here for the phrase 'Hello World.'

Convert the bursts into a numerical scale for phrase HELLO WORLD:

0 = no burst;

1 = an increase or decrease of firing from baseline firing rate;

2 = an increase followed by a decrease below baseline firing rate;

3 = a decrease below baseline firing rate followed by an increase;

4 = an increase followed by a decrease followed by an increase;

5 = a decrease followed by an increase followed by a decrease.

Computers love numbers and decoding loves lots of numbers! So using this classification of bursts, we developed a string of numbers that reflected the bursts and decelerations of activity as the phrase 'Hello World' was spoken. We then used a deep learning approach. The idea is simple: examine the data and select those spoken phrases that have bursts that are the most similar from one phrase to the other. Then select the one typical phrase with a string of numbers that becomes the "target" for the deep learning application. The system will then compare each phrase with the target phrase and see how well they correlate. This is expressed as 'r,' or correlation coefficient (also known as regression). The higher this value is, the higher the correlation. While $r = 1$ would represent a perfect correlation with the target phrase, correlation coefficients of 0.9 or 0.8 are usually considered acceptable. The next figure shows the 'r' for audible speech phrases compared with the target phrase.

Decoding Audible and Silent Speech

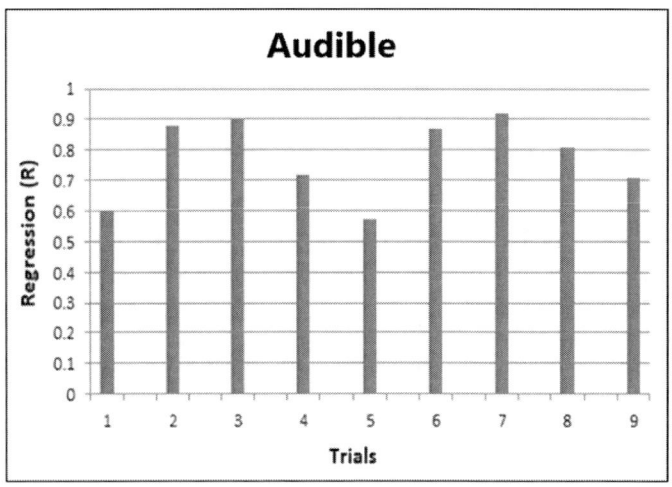

Five of the phrase repetitions had correlations with the target phrase near 0.8 and 0.9. Four had poor correlations: Think of yourself speaking and someone does not understand what you are saying. You will be asked to repeat the phrase and perhaps then the person and you will have a near perfect correlation! Getting low 'r' values does not mean that you cannot repeat what you are saying to get understood.

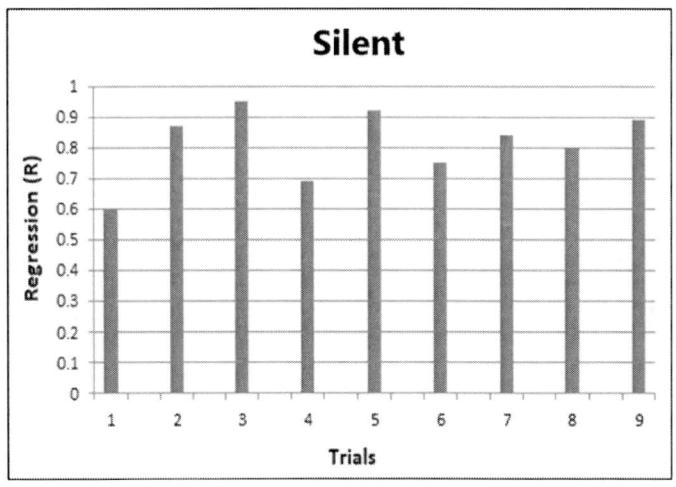

The correlation with the silently spoken phrase was acceptable too, as shown above. Six phrases have an 'r' value between 0.8 and 0.9. This is just as good as the audible data. This was a nice result.

So next, we compared these results with the same decoding program for single units. As you can see in the figure below, the 'r' for the single units was below that for the burst data. And most important of all, the audible and the silent data were not significantly different. Both have similar correlations, 'r', of about 0.6 (remember this is an average!).

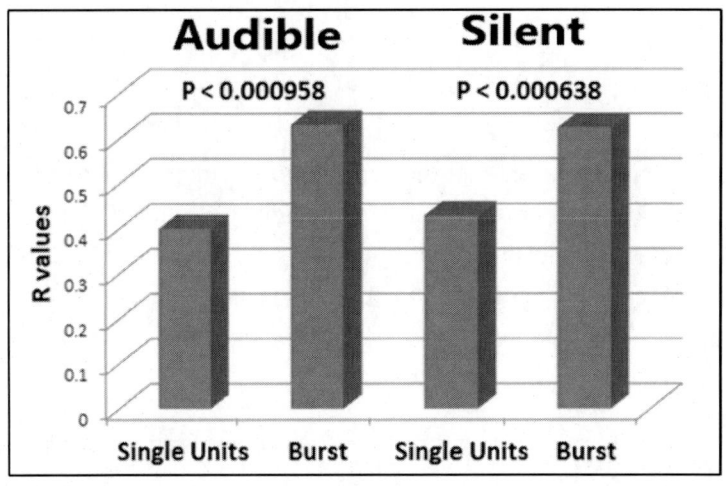

	date	bought	pun	stock	ten	bore	peach	dill	stole	base	bark	scale	skate	scoop	dew	park	got
date	0.91																
bought	0.38	0.93															
pun	0.32	0.4	0.95														
stock	0.27	0.44	0.36	0.97													
ten	0.32	0.32	0.38	0.41	0.94												
bore	0.48	0.43	0.41	0.38	0.51	0.97											
peach	0.35	0.31	0.29	0.27	0.36	0.27	0.92										
dill	0.41	0.32	0.45	0.34	0.38	0.51	0.46	0.94									
stole	0.41	0.38	0.39	0.41	0.39	0.4	0.41	0.39	0.96								
base	0.24	0.32	0.23	0.39	0.27	0.41	0.38	0.4	0.36	0.93							
bark	0.43	0.4	0.46	0.46	0.34	0.44	0.37	0.32	0.38	0.43	0.96						
scale	0.32	0.37	0.39	0.41	0.35	0.39	0.39	0.37	0.36	0.38	0.42	0.96					
skate	0.33	0.34	0.39	0.39	0.41	0.39	0.37	0.37	0.3	0.36	0.33	**0.84**	0.93				
scoop	0.41	0.39	0.29	0.34	0.31	0.34	0.42	0.33	0.38	0.31	0.36	0.32	0.41	0.97			
dew	0.37	0.43	0.51	0.42	0.44	0.46	0.41	0.44	0.38	0.43	0.45	0.42	0.48	0.54	0.96		
park	0.38	0.36	0.42	0.42	0.38	0.47	0.38	0.44	0.42	0.36	<u>0.4</u>	0.42	0.4	0.42	0.42	0.97	
got	0.46	0.32	0.39	0.42	0.37	0.42	0.42	0.35	0.38	0.47	0.38	0.37	0.37	0.36	0.39	0.45	0.99

Decoding Audible and Silent Speech

Recently, we have decoded phones and words. Here is an example of 20 words that have underlying firing rates that are "correlated to themselves" and to the 19 other words. So correlating 'date' to 'date' gives a high correlation of 0.91, but when 'date' is correlated to 'bought' it produces a low correlation of only 0.38. In other words, 'date' can be differentiated from 'bought.'

An example of phones is shown next: The phone 'GUH' was repeated 10 times out loud and 10 times silently. Note the probability value of $p = 0.669$, indicating that there is no difference between Audible and Silent speech. Furthermore, a control period of sitting and not talking or thinking showed a significant difference between the control and both Audible and Silent speech with significant p values less than 0.01.

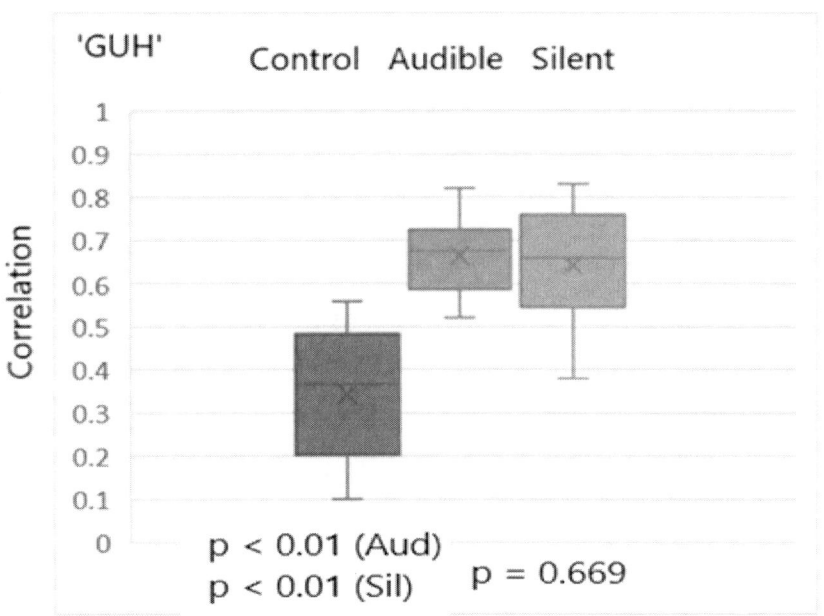

The electrodes and electronics were removed because the incision would not fully close due to the bulk of the electronics. Now that we know how to decode silent speech for phones, words and phrases, and the electrodes have been removed from my brain, what is next?

Chapter 26

THE FUTURE DIRECTION: READY TO IMPLANT LOCKED-IN PEOPLE MORE SUCCESSFULLY?

Well, the obvious answer is to implant locked-in folks who need to speak!

Not so fast! Hold your horses! There are problems.

First, there are not enough signals. We had 65 single units recorded from my brain, which is a respectable number. But many of those were not recognized as being involved in speech decoding. The solution: Four Neurotrophic Electrodes spaced 6 mm apart would cover the speech motor area. And with two pairs of wires in each electrode, there should be 8 pairs times 20 single units, giving us 160 units. This should be plenty. So why not? Because we cannot implant more single channel electronic wireless devices because they are too bulky. So we need more signals and a smaller device. Recall we used single channel implantable systems. We cannot record the 160 single units through an implantable *multichannel* recording system because there is no such implantable recording system yet available. It should be available soon, however.

This brings up another current approach: An alternative is to use a system that exits through the scalp. This is a possibility but raises the question of infection through the opening. And it is temporary, whereas the implantable system and electrodes should be permanent. It is possible to switch the temporary externalized system to the implantable internal system and this is being considered with some trepidation. Infection is a daunting possibility and may damage the person's brain.

The fourth problem is cost. The cost is high even if we go abroad to do the implant (about $30,000 versus $100,000 in the USA), the cost of the external recording system is about $150,000, then there is the need to work with the subject which requires at least two people for about a year (about $200,000) and other computers and software. These things add up. And that is just for one person to learn to speak! However, since implanting Erik in 2004, the National Institutes of Health have realized that getting project from 'bench to bedside' is costly and difficult to fund. So they have developed other funds to do that and we have applied.

Another possible solution is this book: It may be a bestseller! All proceeds, (bestseller or not-so-good seller) will go to a fund to drive this research forward. Erik's family will receive a small percentage of the revenues and the rest will go into the fund. There is also a documentary being produced and scheduled to be released in 2020 that may drive sales of this book. So the obvious thing to do is to set up a 'go fund me' project to raise even more funds with the publicity from this book and documentary.

In summary, when we get past these stumbling blocks the person who is paralyzed and mute will speak again.

Chapter 27

WHY NOT USE OTHER ELECTRODES AND SYSTEMS?

The short answer is: they don't work in the long-term, whereas the Neurotrophic Electrode has documented endurance of a decade in one patient and four years in others. In other words, 85% of their signals are lost in three years [13]. So they won't last long enough for the lifetime of a locked-in person. However, don't get me wrong, they are very effective in the short term. Use of the Utah array, which is supplied by Blackrockneuro.com, has allowed paralyzed subjects to control their paralyzed limbs and feed themselves using a robotic limb or their own paralyzed limb. These electrodes and various computer systems plus sophisticated robotic limbs, have demonstrated a welcome way to restore movement [14, 15].

The problem with these electrodes in the long-term is that *gliosis growth* occurs between the electrode and the brain tissue [13]. Gliosis essentially means the formation of a scar that will always separate the electrode recording tip from the active neural signals. This occurs with all types of electrodes that are simply placed close to neurons, axons or other types of neuropil areas. Recent results with a 3072 tine (or pin) electrode system from Elon Musk's Neuralink that is implanted using a robotic device will likely suffer the same fate of scarring and loss of signal over the long-term, though it attempts to avoid scarring by making the electrodes flexible and small. Nevertheless, the tiny pins will be rejected by the brain, as it has with all other electrodes based on the same principle of operation [13]. We most certainly acknowledge that over the short term the signals look good. These devices with multiple electrodes have and will reveal many more secrets of the central nervous system. However, there is now experimental evidence that the loss of single units allows multi-units to remain that can be analyzed. These multi units can be subjected to training with deep learning AI paradigms. These paradigms allow continuation of the multi-units to act as control signals such that finger movements, for example, can be controlled. How extensive the scarring needs to be before the signals are completely lost is unknown. The question of how long the control endures even with AI paradigms is an issue that will obviously take time to answer.

Other workers [16] are using electrodes placed on the surface of the brain. These are called electrocorticographic recordings (ECOG for short). These signals have been excellent in controlling computers for spelling and detecting spoken phrases [17]. But there is reason to doubt that these electrodes will not be affected by scarring and thus the signals will degrade over time. However, the signals used are in the frequency range and may be less affected by separation of the electrode tips from the brain. As mentioned above, deep learning AI may 'rescue' the signal and allow adequate control to continue. Again, as I wrote above, the question of how long the ECOG signals will endure is an issue that can only be answered over time.

Yet other workers are attempting to use external electroencephalographic signals (EEG for short) to decode speech [19] and control movement [20]. These have been successful in controlling crude movements and detecting simple words, and allied with powerful neural net computing paradigms, may result in more refined movements and more words. However EEG signals have low spatial resolution (they sample from a large cortical territory), and the skull separating the electrode from the brain acts as a filter, letting through only low-frequency components of the brain signals and rejecting the high-frequency components. Combined, these drawbacks are likely to impede their ability to decode speech and impede their ability to produce fine finger movements.

In other labs, Facebook scientists are using Near Infrared (NIR) light to interpret blood flow changes that correlate with neural activity. They expect to detect silent speech using NIR. However, resolution is working against them. Speech at the level of a conversation requires the highest possible resolution and that is only found by recording from single neurons.

So What?

So why do I claim that the Neurotrophic Electrode will survive the lifetime of a person? It all comes down to the hard evidence. As you can read in chapter 12 in part 3, the neural signals at year nine in Erik were successfully subjected to conditioning [2][21]. That implies that they were functional and not some arbitrary noise. We were fortunate to obtain the histological analysis of the tissue inside the electrode that had remained there for 13 years before Erik died. The histology showed neural filaments which are electrically active and, just as important, showed no scarring. These data combined with the recording data imply longevity. [These data are being reviewed for publication [18].]

From a theoretical point of view, the Neurotrophic Electrode ought to work because the active neural signals are carried along axons that are essentially trapped inside the tiny glass cone, as shown in the illustration in the Introduction to part 3. So even if the brain wanted to reject the system, it is held within the brain by the tissue inside the glass cone. The components are all biocompatible: glass, Teflon insulated gold wires and standard surgical glue (methylmethacrylate), as well as the proprietary trophic factors placed inside the cone before implantation.

An occasional objection to the Neurotrophic Electrode is that it records an insufficient number of signals. Yet if this were so, then how could 23 single units be decoded to produce so many phones? How could the 23 single units demonstrate decoding of silent speech [2][22]? There are two reasons: First, just a handful of signals can be conditioned to control the speech

---

[21] See reference summary on page 91.
[22] See reference summary on page 91.

articulators as the evidence above illustrates. Secondly, the present results also imply that thousands of signals are not needed for a prosthetic. They may be needed for basic scientific research, but not for a prosthetic like the one needed for speech synthesis. So more electrodes to collect more and more signals are not critical for the long-term speech prosthetic.

In summary, we have strong evidence that the neural signals from the Neurotrophic Electrode persist over a decade and are functional throughout that time. No other electrode has come close to this achievement and the current evidence indicates they will not. We should thank our fearless colleagues – Marjorie, Johnny, Tim, David and Erik – for without their courage and steadfastness we would not be where we are today!

Chapter 28

THE FUTURE IS ALMOST HERE

See! The winter is past;
the rains are over and gone.
Flowers appear on the Earth.
The season of singing has come.

--- Song of Songs, 2:11 & 12

The demands of scientific research are multi-layered and precise, but often the *need* supported is conceptually simple.

This person's eye has lost its ability to focus. How can we fix that?

This individual is paralyzed and can no longer speak. How can we reclaim her speech?

That person's spinal cord was severed. Can we repair it and still maintain the electrical language of nerves and synapses?

The following areas of new science can help us answer "yes" in these categories!

SPEECH PROSTHETIC

There are 30,000 people suffering with ALS in the USA. After about 4-5 years they get so weak they need a ventilator to breath and stay alive.

Ninety percent decline the ventilator! And yet, many more people will decide to stay on the ventilator once they realize they can speak again because with speech you can converse with family, control your environment and your computer, even run a business on the Internet. There are 15 to 20 times more people worldwide who could be helped with the speech prosthetic. That is 600,000! And they need help.

Brainstem stroke is another group who need the speech prosthetic. It is difficult to come up with a definite number, but there are approximately 50,000 brainstem stroke persons (like Erik) in the USA. They need it too. So that is 1,000,000 worldwide.

For them, the future is almost here!

MOVEMENT PROSTHETIC

The future for other severely handicapped people is bright. For those with paralysis of limbs, there is a justifiable expectation that they will control their limbs again, either crudely through external devices (such as EEG), or if fine finger movements are desired, by implanting that part of the brain that once did control the fingers. Magnetic resonant images show that the finger control part of the cortex is still alive even though they cannot move! The American Paralysis association tells us that there are 125,000 quadriplegics in the USA. That adds up to 2,500,000 worldwide! They need a long-term electrode whose signals drive muscle stimulation devices, or that control a robotic limb.

This technology applies to those with conditions such as damage to their axons as they exit the spinal cord (axonal neuropathy), and those who have muscular dystrophy so they are almost paralyzed or fully paralyzed and must sit in a wheelchair to gain any mobility.

Talking about wheelchairs, there is no reason to doubt that the cortical control signals can be collared into double duty: Not just controlling a paralyzed limb but also controlling a wheelchair.

In fact, why not use these control signals to control an *exoskeleton*, a form-fitting body suit whose joints are motorized. Soldiers use these suits to carry large loads while running on the battlefield. Quite amazing! So why not put them on a paralyzed person, such as someone with ALS or quadriplegia, who can use the cortical control signals recorded through the electrodes to operate the exoskeleton? That is being done right now.

Say you want to upgrade the quality of the moment? How about environmental controls such as TV, music, Internet, computer and so on. Sure, these can be accessed with a switch or EEG, but once the electrodes are implanted why not put their signals to other uses, too?

FUTURISTIC USAGES

Let's go even further:

How about augmenting your brain power? Don't be surprised if I tell you, you already do. Look at your cell phone or computer: Go ahead – open Google or open Wikipedia. All the information you will ever need and more is right there! Open your cell phone and ask Siri a question. Ask Alexa a question. See, you have more information at your fingers than anyone ever had before on this earth. Need a calculator? Got it! On your phone or computer. Need to contact someone in a hurry? Call them on your phone. In less of a hurry? Text them. Even less of a hurry, then email them. So you have already augmented your brain power! You can be informed, can calculate faster and can communicate like no one on earth has ever done before!

CAN WE GO FURTHER STILL?

Yes! And here is where we can push the boundaries even further: Why not augment normal brain function with Neurotrophic Electrodes implanted in 'normal people'? If, and it is a big if, we could connect to appropriate parts of the brain we could upgrade the ability to communicate, inform and calculate.

To communicate, you'd simply implant a miniature 'hearing aid' inside the ear to receive a phone call, and then while speaking silently (of course) record the neural signals from the speech cortex and transmit them from an imbedded transmitter to whoever called you. Yes, I realize that is not feasible now, but with miniaturization it may be possible.

Need to look something up or use a calculator? You just use the information that reside in the 'cloud.' The 'cloud' is essentially composed of massive data storage banks here on mother earth! To send requests, we speak silently and transmit what we say as a text message request to the cloud. To receive info from the 'cloud,' content could be transmitted to the 'hearing aid' embedded in the ear.

FUTURE SHOPPING

Think of going shopping. You buy a device to allow you to communicate silently, such as a cell phone *implanted in* your brain. Then go to the local neurosurgeon to get it robotically implanted. Done deal! For your 21st birthday, instead of getting breast implants, your parents buy you a gift of the system that communicates with the cloud. Then you trot back down to your friendly surgeon who supervises it being robotically implanted.

I know that is not possible now, but it may be one day. Never doubt technology when fueled by the imagination!

KNOWING AND DOING!

Futuristic usages raise ethical problems. First and foremost, is who gets the augmentation? Nefarious governments and equally nefarious private armies will want to augment their troops and police. How to stop that? Make the system available to all. Too expensive for Joe Soap? Yes, at first. But the cost of technology always comes down. Once it does come down, then everyone has a chance to avail of it, augment themselves as they wish – if we set in motion now the intention to offer these breakthroughs to all levels of society. The rich will always have their new toys, so let's make sure everyone else can sign up for what they need from new tech as well! Knowing the right thing to do should lead to doing the right thing! *Right?*

Chapter 29

SCIENTIFIC COMMENTARIES

ANDRE JOEL CERVANTES

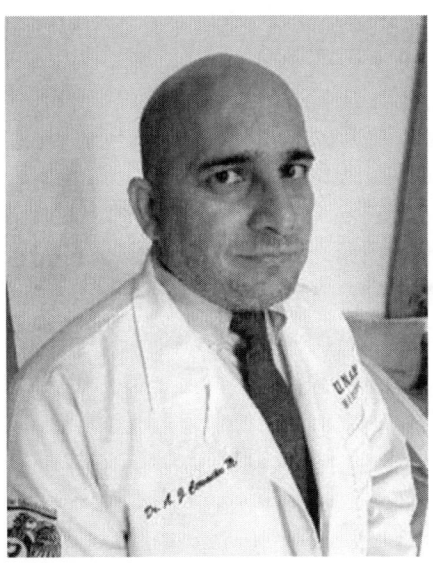

Andre Joel Cervantes, neurosurgeon, Belize City, Belize. He trained in medicine and neurosurgery at the National Autonomous University of Mexico (UNAM) in Mexico City. He now practices in Belize and Mexico. Areas of special interest include Functional, Stereotactic, Radio and Spine Surgery. He co-founded the Belize International Institute of Neuroscience, he founded the Neurosurgical and Spinal Services Associates and is president of the Belize Society of Neurological Surgeons. He has co-authored several scientific papers.

Commentary

The Road to Lunacy?

There are things one embarks on with a full sense of purpose, and other things we venture into not really ever knowing why. On balance, I would say I am the fortunate one, the one who has gotten away with it all. My trips to "Lunacy" have not been without a smile or two.

While a neurosurgical resident I discovered the fascinating world of Functional, Stereotactic and Radio Neurosurgery where one learns to modulate brain functions in very sick people who otherwise would have no solution with conventional Neurosurgery, Neurology and Psychiatry.

One reads, loses him or herself in what our mentors are doing and saying on a regular basis. Actually I remember one such mentor whom as a resident I never really met but was utterly fascinated by his scientific approach to things. I guess growing up as a kid in my native country Belize everything we ever knew about television was WGN, a station in Chicago Illinois. Naturally I had a positive bias towards Chicagoans and everything Chicago. A Dr. Roy Bakay M.D., FAANS (RIP) from Rush University in Chicago was silently one of my mentors while I was a neurosurgical resident in Mexico City.

I completed Neurosurgical Residency and Fellowships both in Spinal Surgery and Functional, Stereotactic and Radio Neurosurgery in 2005. I returned home as my country's first Neurosurgeon and settled down to the challenging task of educating my Belizean society about the benefits and necessity of establishing a strong neurosurgical practice and presence in Belize. It soon became a realization there would be no governmental or private enterprise support for my level of training, which was viewed as light years ahead of what Belize should be prepared to have to serve its citizens.

I centered my energies on the practice of General Neurosurgery with focuses on Neurotrauma, Neuro Intensive Care, and Spine Surgery and, curiously, in less than 6 months, I found myself working some specialized areas of Clinical Neurology and Neuropsychiatry. While my background in Functional, Stereotactic and Radio Neurosurgery was fulfilling needs in key areas in my Belizean society, there was nevertheless, a subtle emptiness, a feeling of something lacking. Were I to be totally honest, I felt, I missed miserably being able to offer neuromodulation brain and spine surgery. It was a struggle because I so badly wanted to stay home versus wanting to go back to one of those highly-advanced neurosurgical practices that continually courted my steps to leave Belize. I tend to be a determined dreamer, so I decided to stay and prayed and prayed that this decision was the right one.

One day I received an email from a US-based (Neuroscientist/Neurologist) Dr. Philip Kennedy and a Dr. Roy Bakay (Functional and Stereotactic Neurosurgeon)!!!! I was in utter disbelief. I quickly accepted to receive them in my country for a friendly talk. How could my silent mentor (Dr. Bakay) be coming to see me? He was a man I had never personally met, and why would he come to see me?

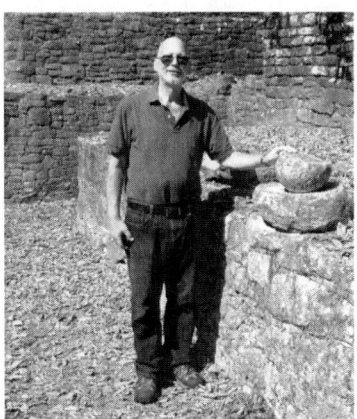

On the anointed day I met a deflated version of Dr. Bakay, and I quickly realized my mentor was not in the best of health. Dr. Bakay was mostly silent beyond silent. His silence spoke volumes on his declining health.

Dr. Philip Kennedy was soft spoken and displayed a very assertive character. It impacted me to see my mentor relatively silent but his companion filled me in quite easily as to the purpose of their visit. "Oh" I thought, "Professor Bakay and Dr. Philip Kennedy have come to explore an option or two."

The following day I had a quiet talk alone with Dr. Kennedy. We agreed to call each other just "Phil" and "Joel". Phil turned out to be as down-to-earth a guy as Roy was. He explained that Roy had an end stage condition, and, also faced FDA constraints for certain experimental neurosurgical procedures to be done on human subjects in the USA. They had come to Belize to try their luck with me. I agreed to assist Professor Bakay in his endeavors.

It wasn't long after that we received a locked-in patient (Erik) from the USA for placement of motor speech brain electronics, a "first" for the country of Belize.

I remember scrubbing in to assist Dr. Bakay and reflecting on this kind of-a-first-time-surgery in Belize. I had placed many brain and spinal cord Electrodes in training before, but never the opportunity for this type of experimental brain electronics. Truly a first for me!

To my surprise Professor Bakay asked for me to do the surgery which I gladly accepted. For a moment, I felt the eyes of the entire operating suite personnel, the neurosurgical world and the entire nation of Belize on me. Oh Lord! Would I be able to pull this off?

Settling my nerves, I focused on the task at hand and ventured into my world. I actually forgot that "I was being observed" and applied myself to doing this surgery as best as possible, because in fact, I had a very needful human being in front of me who was depending on the skill of my hands and my decision-making processes to obtain a much better quality of life.

Surgery was uneventful and deemed a success by myself, Phil and Roy. In fact, I was amazed that Roy had little to no participation while Phil had a much more active participation coaching along the placement of the electronics. Then it dawned on me that these two gentlemen were indeed the consummate professionals I had deemed them to be. That day I adopted them both as my mentors. I remember going back to review Phil's curriculum vitae and really taking an in-depth look at it, much more than I had done initially.

And then I understood, Roy was dying... and dying soon and Phil needed to carry on these projects alone. A silence overtook my soul. Could I take on this responsibility?

Then I had a flashback about the OR setting, Roy had looked at Phil and said something under his breath while nodding. I presume it meant I had passed the test. Equally important, it was also the passing of the baton from Roy to Phil.

It wasn't long after that that Roy passed away back home in the USA and I was left to correspond with Phil. I quickly decided that Phil is really one of these soft spoken heavyweight fighters who puts all their knockout power in the ring. There is no way you can tell him "no" once he has entered that ring.

Life throws many sliders and curve balls at you, not everything is a homerun. As the plans and months passed by, Phil was never off the radar and communicated frequently. Potential candidates for surgery popped up and then withdrew. Then, out of the blue Phil asked me if I would consider placing brain Electrodes *in his own brain*.

This is where lunacy meets and marries lunacy!!!! A "yes" answer was not hard to give. Phil puts a special energy on everything. He has a direct and practical route to everything he does but life and neurosurgery is not always such a direct path. Sometimes "the long way around the barn is the shortest way home!"

I have insomnia when I am ultra-excited about something that I am passionate about. I have thanked life, God and the universe for meeting and working with Phil and his unique subjects. My insomnia was not ever about if I should or should not operate on Phil, that was understood. What fueled my curiosity and hunger was the thought of being able to partake in finding out how, when, what normal speech motor neurons did to communicate.

When Phil returned to Belize, he came alone! No relative or friend to accompany him on this Star Wars adventure. Ha ha ha...very much Phil now that I know him better. Our medical team leader was alarmed. The night before surgery, I spoke with the pillows, life, God and the universe. Then I calmed my fears and tamed my demons with some intoxicatingly melodic ballads from the likes of Scorpions and Metallica just to name a few.

The day of surgery Phil looked me in the eyes and said "Roy and I have never doubted your capabilities. You can do this Joel." That ultra-boosted my confidence and I know Roy was with me and has been with me ever since.

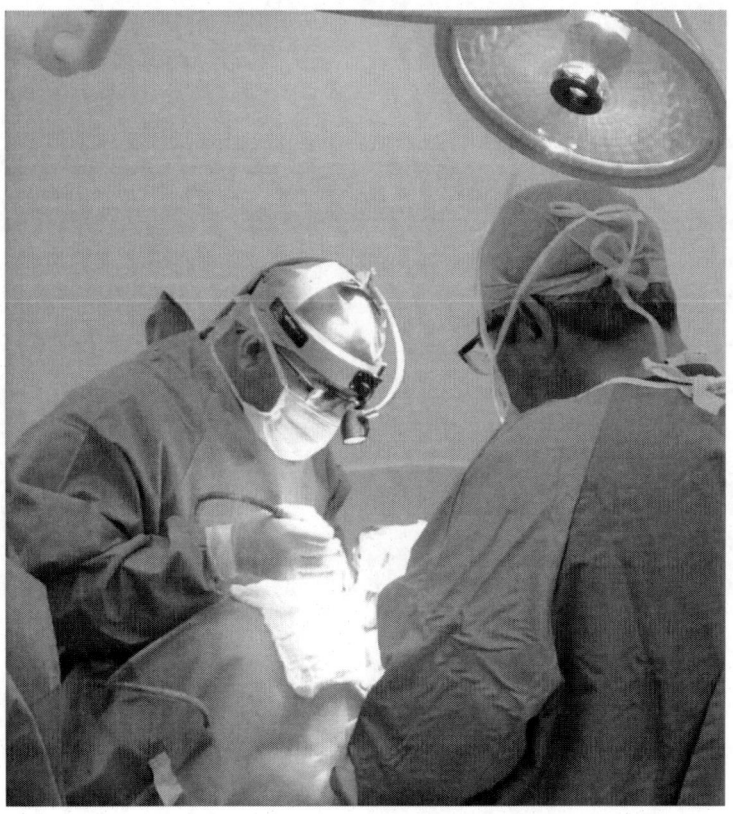

My anesthesiologists had always known I was missing several screws but that day they proved I could never come back to any sense of normalcy. I remember well each step with the obsessions of a type seen only in the spying of a jealous wife. I am known to be very careful and precise in all my consults and surgeries. But I am also known to be extremely daring. I would not be writing this piece today without having such a volatile and intoxicating psychic mix.

That day I married my God to my demons in the operating suite, and got away with it, or so I have thought. Looking at Phil's brain I remembered wondering if I should be looking for macroscopic signs of the dementia changes in his brain that brought him to this! How could he have entrusted a neurosurgeon to place Electrodes in a normal brain?

My conclusion has been we are both not of this world, we are two outcasts who dream in expanding the universes of neuroscience. As I stared down at Phil's brain, closing my eyes a couple of seconds to breathe and suck it all in, I remembered Roy's legacy and then it happened... A few seconds later I was asking my support team to hand me what I needed to close. It was done! Brain Electrodes had been placed on a genius and a lunatic in a beautiful little country called Belize, all while an esteemed, recently passed neurosurgeon and a band of angels looked on!

Phil's postoperative course was not without minor setbacks. He temporarily developed focal motor seizures of his jaw and had to be chaperoned back home by his son. He did not however develop midterm complications, and long term complications have as yet to arise. Unfortunately a scalp infection necessitated for the Electrodes and electronics to be removed a couple of months after I placed them. In between, I can imagine Phil sitting in his lab recording neural signals from his own brain, each session a special gift and opportunity.

Phil is a friend, a mentor, a lunatic, a philanthropist, a son of this universe and a consummate neuroscientist. Phil is proof of the ultimate sacrifice a living human being can do. He has been really kind to include me as a coauthor in several papers and posters. He and Roy have helped me to make history in my beautiful little jewel of a country known as Belize.

I think anyone would agree that the fathers of modern intraoperative neuromodulation brain surgery in Belize are Phil, Roy and myself. I welcome other Philip Kennedys and Roy Bakays to help the scientific world grow neuroscience, neurology, neuropsychiatry and neurosurgery for the benefit of mankind. Belize is ideally legislated for this type of development especially in the world of Functional and Stereotactic Neurosurgery.

I say this with the utmost pride: "thanks to you, Phil and Roy". Thanks Phil for keeping the light of brain and spine neuromodulation burning deep inside of me. At the same time, Phil knows he can continue depending on me as the need arises.

PROFESSOR EBERHARD FETZ

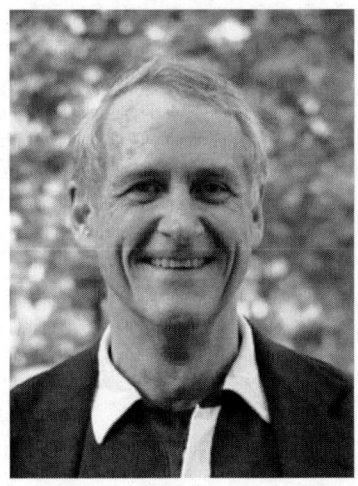

Eberhard Fetz received his Ph.D. in physics from the Massachusetts Institute of Technology in 1967. He is currently Professor in the Department of Physiology & Biophysics and DXARTS, with an adjunct appointment in Bioengineering. He is a Core Staff member in the Washington National Primate Research Center and Thrust Leader (for Experimental Neuroscience) in the Center for Neurotechnology, Seattle, Washington.

Commentary

His overall research has concerned the neural control of limb movement in primates and mechanisms of neural computation. This began with studies of monkeys' ability to volitionally control the activity of brain cells. In this operant conditioning paradigm monkeys controlled a biofeedback meter arm with patterns of activity in motor cortex neurons. This work in 1969 first showed that neural activity could be used to drive an external device, and demonstrated the ability of the brain to volitionally control the activity of individual and multiple cortical neurons in variable patterns, phenomena that underlie much of the current work in brain-machine interfaces. He went on to investigate the functional organization of motor cortex cells controlling forearm muscles by documenting the correlational linkages of output cells with muscles in spike-triggered averages of EMG. He pioneered the recording of spinal interneurons in behaving monkeys and showed that spinal neurons share many properties of cortical cells, including preparatory activity prior to instructed movements. Other studies investigated the synaptic interactions between cortical neurons by using *in vivo* intracellular recordings and spike-triggered averages of membrane potentials. To elucidate neural computations in large-scale neural networks he developed dynamic recurrent network models that simulate the neural interactions generating behavior like target tracking and short-term memory; recent work modeled the neural mechanisms underlying cortical plasticity. Most recently, his lab has developed an implantable recurrent brain-computer chip interface that can record activity of cortical cells during free behavior and convert this activity in real time to stimulation of cortex, spinal cord or muscles. This so-called "neurochip" creates a continuously operating artificial feedback loop that the brain can learn to incorporate into behavior. A second application of the neurochip is to produce changes in the strength of synaptic connections through activity-dependent stimulation. The synaptic mechanisms underlying these plastic changes in motor cortical connections were captured in neural network models that made important testable predictions.

The demonstration that neural activity can be volitionally controlled raises some interesting issues. Our early studies showed that monkeys could readily increase and decrease activity of single motor cortex neurons when that activity drove the deflection of a neurofeedback meter arm to a level that consistently triggered a feeder. Monkeys could quickly learn to change the activity patterns of neurons and muscles to drive the meter to threshold and so get reward. Surprisingly, they could produce multiple orthogonal patterns in the course of a single session. And consistent correlations between cells and muscles could be dissociated when such dissociation was explicitly rewarded.

Volitional control of motor cortex neurons is easy to understand because these neurons are normally involved in activating muscles. However, there is increasing evidence that activity of cells in many non-motor regions of the brain can also be volitionally controlled. Neurons in areas that have been traditionally thought to be involved in sensory functions nevertheless have central drive as well. Cells in sensory cortices that are reliably driven by "bottom-up" peripheral input can also be modulated by "top-down" volitional input. This has now been demonstrated in primary somatosensory [where sensory stimuli are detected] and visual cortices. Neurons involved in internal "thinking" are also clearly controllable. As explored in Phil Kennedy's study of Erik, the neurons involved in generating speech are a particularly important group of volitionally controllable neurons for speech prostheses.

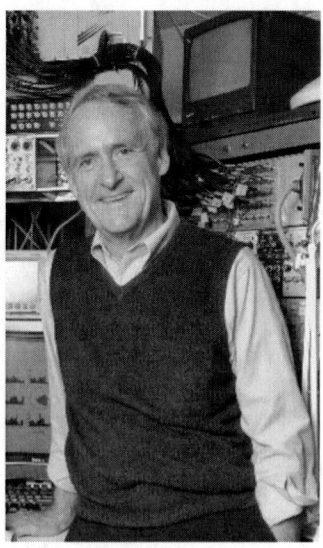

In some cases the number of neurons recorded simultaneously are relatively few, raising the question: how much can the activity of a few neurons be leveraged to control multiple dimensions of an external device? To what extent do increasing numbers of neurons add greater control? As first shown by Humphrey et al and Carmena, Nicolelis et al, the ability to extract different movement parameters from the same population of cells increases with the number of task-related neurons included. Given the freedom to optimize the transform between firing rates of a population and the controlled variables, one could assume that additional units can only serve to increase control, because the transform algorithm would ignore the activity of any neurons that don't improve control. However, for a specific behavior, the incremental addition in control for each neuron would tend to decrease with the total number due to redundancy. However, a significant factor here is the number of behavioral conditions that need to be controlled; the more different conditions, the more will additional units be helpful.

Another important factor for success with BCIs is the amount of time available for learning control. The mechanisms of learning BCI control are similar to mechanisms for learning new motor behaviors. The brain is remarkably flexible in devoting neurons to sensory and motor tasks, even to the extent of crossing sensory modalities. The phenomenon of sensory substitution shows that under appropriate circumstances the brain can interpret spatiotemporal patterns of somatic stimulation in terms of "visual" spatial perception. Thus, the higher-order areas mediating spatial perception can readily switch from using visual to somatic information. The critical factors here include an active motor-sensory loop; for example, the ability to control the camera whose images are converted to somatic stimulation. Similarly, in the motor system there is an analogous ability to flexibly connect motor planning to execution. Neurons used to achieve a goal in a BCI context may initially be driven by appropriate cognitive imagery, but are eventually driven by the intension to achieve the goal.

An interesting issue raised by brain control of neural activity is the nature of the controller. Presumably the neural networks involved in generating volitional control are distributed in higher-order areas of the brain. These circuits develop through active interaction with the peripheral world, leading to a representation of an autonomous self. The perception of self is remarkably robust, yet relatively little is known about the underlying neural mechanisms, compared to mechanisms of sensory and motor representations. This internal perception of 'self' survives sensory loss and motor paralysis, as shown by the continuing ability to volitionally control neural activity. Does this 'self' disappear in the fully locked-in patient who has no ability to interact with the world, or does it still persist, as maintained by Niels Birbaumer? The ability to express itself through BCIs surely makes a huge difference in maintaining the 'self'. So beyond communication, the effect on survival of 'self' is another reason that BCI work will continue to be important. [As elucidated in chapter 6, "The place where "I" exists".]

PROFESSOR ANDREW JACKSON

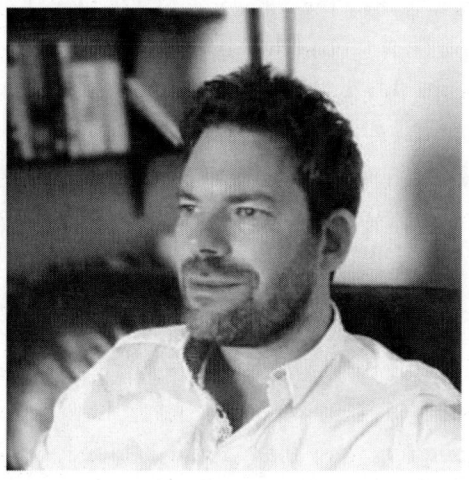

Andrew Jackson is a Professor of Neural Interfaces and a Wellcome Trust Senior Research Fellow at the Institute of Neuroscience, Newcastle University, UK. After studying at Oxford University (Physics) and University College London (Neuroscience), Andrew worked for four years with Prof Eberhard Fetz at the University of Washington, Seattle, developing new technologies for bidirectional brain interfaces. Since 2006 he has led a laboratory at Newcastle addressing fundamental scientific questions relating to the control of movement, neural dynamics, sleep and learning. This basic research informs the development of new closed-loop neural interface therapies for conditions including stroke, spinal cord injury and epilepsy.

Commentary

There are a number of patient groups that could benefit in future from brain interfaces, such as people with spinal cord injury or amputees. But there are already many other assistive technologies that can help these people in their daily lives. This sets quite a high bar for how well an interface needs to work in order to really benefit the user in practice - a prosthetic limb that is well-controlled by the stump is better than one that is badly-controlled by the brain. I think the difference with the locked-in condition is how few alternatives there are for these people to communicate. This means that even a cumbersome interface that doesn't work 100% of the time can make a huge difference to people's lives. Of course, what we really want is a convenient interface that works all of the time, and these days there is a lot of hype about the future of brain interfaces. But I think the pioneering work that Dr. Kennedy and others have done with locked-in people really demonstrated the reality of how brain interfaces have the power to change lives now.

My own view on whether non-invasive techniques can provide conversational speech is that there are huge challenges for brain interfacing using non-invasive techniques, but also huge opportunities. It's often been said that trying to read the brain from the scalp is like trying to work out what's happening on the football pitch by standing outside the stadium and listening to the roar of the crowd. I'm not sure we've seen really substantial improvements in electroencephalography (EEG) interfaces in recent years, which may suggest we're close to the limit of the information that can be extracted from electrical fields at the scalp. However, there are some exciting possibilities in alternative modalities. Wearable magnetoencephalography (MEG) has been coming along nicely – whereas we used to need large, super-cooled machinery to detect magnetic fields from the brain, this can now be done by small, room-temperature sensors. DARPA's new 'Next-Generation Nonsurgical Neurotechnology' programme is funding a wide range of new techniques from injectable nanotransducers to acousto-optical imaging techniques. At the same time, companies like Facebook, OpenWater, etc. are investing heavily in their own ideas. It's too early to say what approach will prove most successful, but I wouldn't want to bet against seeing some radical breakthroughs in the next few years.

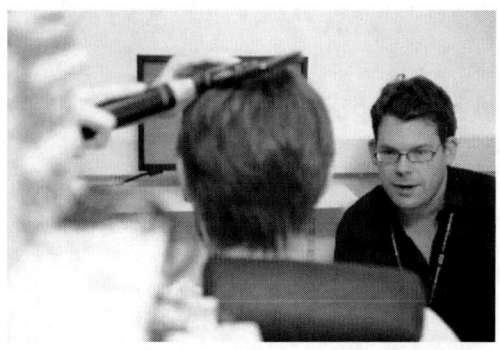

Having said that, there is also a lot of investment in new types of invasive interfaces, for example with Elon Musk's Neuralink grabbing headlines at the moment. High-density arrays, like the NeuroPixels probe, that have integrated microelectronics and hundreds or thousands of channels on a single hair-like shaft have changed the way we do neuroscience research and may soon be tested in humans. Again it's hard to know which will prove successful but it is certainly an interesting time for the field.

When we think about current AI and neural net paradigms enhancing our data decoding I think a good historical analogy might be with speech recognition software. Neural interfaces are perhaps around where we were in the 1980s with computer systems that had to be trained for many hours to recognise a single speaker, and even then got about half of the words wrong. Today Amazon will sell you something for your mantelpiece that can understand the voice of anyone who comes round to visit. Is it possible to conceive of a similar trajectory for neural interfaces? On the one hand there is still a lot we don't understand about how the brain represents and processes thoughts. We don't really know how language is encoded, especially at a level more abstract than the direct motor commands heading out to the muscles. Currently in the neuroscience there's a lot of focus on what David Marr called the 'implementation' level – engineering advances are allowing us to record more and more channels of neural signals but we've yet to make as much progress in understanding representations, computations etc. On the other hand, 1980s linguists were probably also arguing that we needed to better understand the high-level structure of language before we could make progress with speech recognition. In fact what happened was that the increasing availability of large datasets and sophisticated machine learning techniques rendered a lot of that unnecessary.

As we develop better neural interface technology, we may get to a stage where the datasets are large enough to apply similar approaches, in which we don't worry too much about the science and just let machine learning figure it out. As a neuroscientist, I find it a slightly depressing thought - that we may in future be able to build workable brain-machine interfaces without making any further progress in our understanding of how the brain works (but I guess we should all be worried about losing our jobs to artificial intelligence).

As a side note, I think the field of neuroscience is uniquely at risk of a whole lot of conceptual confusion when it comes to machine learning. Artificial neural networks are getting incredibly powerful and can model almost any complex system from the stock markets to hurricanes. But economists and meteorologists are unlikely to confuse the nodes in their networks with actual share certificates or rain droplets. By contrast, when we model the neural networks in our brains using artificial neural networks in a computer, we need to be very careful about how far we push the interpretation of these models.

Anyway, it is undoubtedly true that machine learning will prove extremely useful for decoding neural data. But the traditional 'supervised' approaches rely on large amounts of labelled data, e.g., using pictures that a human has already identified as a house or a car to train a network to recognise more houses and cars in future. When it comes to brain decoding, it is harder to know where all these labels will come from. How far can we really get by instructing people to think about specific things, or asking them afterwards what they were thinking about? Some of the work that I think is most exciting is applying 'unsupervised' approaches that look for higher-level structure in brain data - if we can find this structure then it may map in a more meaningful way onto the structure of thoughts. This gives me some hope for neuroscience too, because these structures should also provide us with insights into the workings of the brain.

Finally, with all the excitement of machine learning, we shouldn't forget that we are talking about connecting to a neural network with more capabilities and far more creativity than anything that Google has yet made – the human brain! So let's try not forget the brain's ability to learn in all this. I've often said that we should think of neural interfaces not as prosthetics that replace some part of the nervous system, but as tools that we can learn to use to do what we want. Ultimately, we need to find a creative synthesis between human and machine learning to really maximize the potential of these technologies.

THOMAS WICHMANN

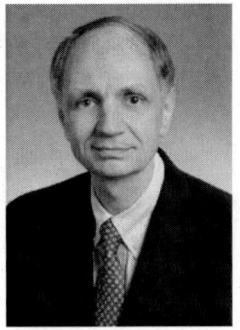

Dr. Wichmann received medical training in Germany, followed by postdoctoral training in pharmacology and electrophysiology at the University of Freiburg (Germany) and Johns Hopkins University (Baltimore, MD). In the early 1990s, he completed residency training in Neurology at Emory University (Atlanta, GA), and has been a professor in the movement disorder division in the Department of Neurology at the same

University since then, specializing in research and treatment of Parkinson's disease and Huntington's disease. His research focuses on brain activity changes that are associated with Parkinson's disease, and the effects of DBS on brain networks. His work has been continuously funded by NIH and private foundations, and has been published in high-impact journals, such as *Science, Brain, Nature* and *Journal of Neuroscience*.

Commentary

This book tells a remarkable story. There is a group of patients recently rendered unable to communicate by a brutal medical misfortune. There is a new therapy involving special equipment with the potential to translate their brain's activity into speech. And there is the physician who manages their care, whose passion for realizing this potential leads him to undergoing the therapy himself.

I have for many years been following this story, with all of its surprising twists and turns. The physician, Dr. Phil Kennedy, and I went through residency training in neurology together, and Phil had talked with me even then about his hopes for this new therapy. So, when he asked me to contribute a commentary to his book, I readily agreed. What follows is a compilation of my thoughts about this story, and about Dr. Kennedy's unique position in the field of brain-machine interface development.

Brain-Machine Interfaces

All brain functions, including thoughts and emotions, involve electrical signals that are generated in the brain. To produce behavior, these brain signals are normally sent to the body's muscles via nerves, to induce coordinated activations of groups of muscles commensurate with the desired activity. Speech is an especially complex example: Seemingly we 'dream up' a sentence in our mind which then emerges from our mouth a split-second later. Biologically, this miraculous link between our mind and our behavior corresponds to the generation of highly complex patterns of electrical signals in the brain that are then sent to vocal cords and muscles of the mouth and throat.

In coordination with numerous other muscles of the chest and abdomen that control the air pressure in the lungs, these muscle activations are used to generate communication sounds. The idea that it ought to be possible to build a brain-machine interface with which one could *record* electrical brain signals and use them to control external machines (like a computer) instead of muscles is the foundation of the story told here. Applied to speech, this would mean to use brain signal to control an external speech-synthesizing device.

Such a technique could be especially life-changing for 'locked-in' patients, those whose muscles no longer respond to signals from the brain after a stroke, or because of a disease like amyotrophic lateral sclerosis (ALS). People afflicted with these diseases can literally not move a muscle, and therefore cannot speak, gesture, or signal in any. For them, a speech-centered brain-machine interface would be life-changing, because it would restore their ability to communicate with those around them.

Unfortunately, there is a tremendous chasm between 'ought to be possible' (see above) and current reality. Many years of research and numerous engineering advances have brought us closer, but many staggering challenges still remain before brain-machine interfaces that enable patients to live relatively normal lives can be realized.

Dr. Kennedy's book gives us a chance to join him on this ongoing research journey. It is a measure of his dedication and that of his patients that although neither side is likely to see the final product of the research work in their lifetime, both press on, certain that no progress toward the goal can be made without continuing efforts.

Technical Challenges

The first step in harnessing the electrical signals of the brain to control machines is to record the signals. One of the technically simplest method to achieve this is to obtain recordings of electroencephalographic signals (EEGs). This can be done without surgery and requires only the attachment of wire Electrodes to the skin overlying the skull which are then attached to amplifiers and other equipment. Unfortunately, EEG signals are of very limited use in brain machine interface technology, because it is difficult to know precisely which locations in the brain give rise to which signals, and only very low-frequency signal components can be recorded. EEG signals simply don't provide the information needed to control fast processes like speech.

These limitations can be overcome by using recordings done with Electrodes that are actually inserted into the brain. As Dr. Kennedy describes, it was shown decades ago through research with animals that subjects equipped with such Electrodes can in fact learn to modulate the activity of nerve cells in their brains to earn a reward by controlling a computer or robotic device.

Implanting such Electrodes in human patients though involves more challenges. For one thing, most types of Electrodes simply don't last very long in the brain. The story told here became possible because of Phil's invention of a new type of Electrode, the "Neurotrophic Electrode", which can survive much longer in the brain.

Compared to other devices, however, the Neurotrophic Electrode poses a different challenge in that it is more limited in the number of cells it can record from, and therefore the amount of information that it can collect at any given time. Some ways to get around this problem include implanting a larger number of Electrodes, along with amplifiers that can handle a larger number of channels.

Another challenge is the need to connect the implanted devices to external equipment. Using connectors that penetrate the skin over the skull results in brain signal recordings of high-fidelity, but the skin around the connector is vulnerable to infection and mechanical damage, both of which limit how long the device can be kept in place.

Dr. Kennedy chose instead to implant an amplifier along with the Electrodes into the patient. The amplifier is equipped with a radio wave transmitter that is used to send the brain signals to external equipment. The device is powered wirelessly by an inductive energy transfer system (similar to what can be used to charge some smartphones).

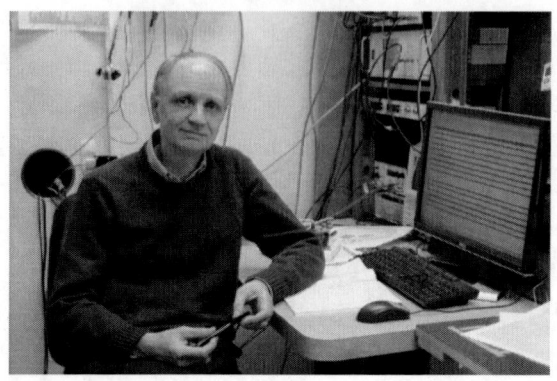

Dr. Kennedy has achieved remarkable successes with his brain-machine interfaces: He has inspired patients to participate as subjects in his research, led the teams that successfully implanted the devices (initially working with his long-term collaborator, the late neurosurgeon, Dr. Roy Bakay), obtained recordings from the devices implanted in the patients, and did painstaking analyses of the data produced by these recordings. It is important to recognize that, besides performing the surgery in his patients, Dr. Kennedy did almost all of the work personally, with very little help from others, because few people have the patience and tenacity necessary to persevere when the challenges are so great and the goal so distant. He remains focused on the tremendous value of the goal of restoring speech for patients who are trapped inside their bodies and does whatever it takes to move toward that goal.

Ethical Questions

Besides the enormous technical challenges of Dr. Kennedy's work, it involves equally daunting challenges in an entirely different realm, that of ethics. At first glance, with physician-researchers eager to carry out their brain-machine interface research and desperate patients eager to participate, it seems that there should be few if any ethical issues to worry about in this kind of research. However, on closer examination, there are subtleties that complicate things considerably. One is that the consent of the patient is clearly necessary before it can be ethical to implant a device into the patient's brain, and then record signals from it. But the very nature of the problem that makes these patients desperate for a solution is that it is difficult or impossible for locked-in patients to communicate anything, including their consent or refusal to grant it, and it is almost impossible to establish that they are (legally and medically) competent to give the consent even if it were known that they are willing to do so. This means that legal consent has to be obtained from family members who speak on the patient's behalf. But many patients who qualify medically to participate in this research find themselves in this state because of a sudden, unexpected event (such as a stroke due to a pontine hemorrhage), having had no chance to provide their family members with clear guidance about their wishes with regard to participation in such research.

The fact that the patients and their families are desperate for help also complicates matters: it may make them less than able to exercise their judgement about risks, and they may simply not hear explanations that the planned research will help to collect data and contribute to the effort, but is not likely to produce the relief for which they yearn. For example, if data from 150 neurons would be needed to effectively govern a speech-synthesizing device, but signals from only 5 neurons can be gathered now from a single participant in the research, the signals from those 5 neurons may be of great value to the research effort, but the patients and their families have to be made to understand that this will not suffice to improve the lives of the current research subjects.

It almost goes without saying that part of the contract made between researchers and patients is that the very best technology will be used, and that strong analysis techniques and statistical methods are in place to guarantee that the available information will be used to its maximal extent. Given the fact that very few patients can participate in research such as described in this book, neither the equipment used, nor the data generated, should be proprietary so that experiments can be repeated by (or can be done in collaboration with) other researchers. Utmost methodological transparency is an important and often overlooked component of the ethical contract with the patient as it determines how impactful the technology can be in the future and which value it ultimately has for all participants, including those who participate in the research.

Patients and their families who agree to participate in research, fully aware of what they are signing up for, are the true heroes in this story. They bear the risks for the sake of benefits they hope to secure for future generations of patients. Their participation is, of course, not entirely without benefit to themselves, but the benefits may be largely intangibles, such as the thrill of being among the few who can contribute to this exciting research adventure, or the reward of interacting regularly with researchers who clearly care deeply about the challenge they face. Phil has a gift for reaching out to patients and letting them know what an integral role they have in this research enterprise that is larger than all of them together.

The ethics of studying or using brain-machine interfaces include another facet as well. Besides using output from the brain to control external devices (the focus of Dr. Kennedy's work), there is also the possibility of using external devices or interventions to alter brain function. The latter is already an important part of common clinical therapies. For example, deep brain stimulation is an effective treatment for otherwise intractable Parkinson's disease. As a reversible treatment for brain disorders that are recognized as devastating, this use is ethically relatively unproblematic. But Dr. Kennedy also touches on the use of 'brain enhancement' for *healthy* individuals, another potential field of development for brain-machine interface technology. We already accept without much thought, many ways of enhancing normal brain function: Up to now, these mostly involve chemicals such as caffeine, alcohol, nicotine, or medications, such as benzodiazepines, that are used to modulate cognitive or emotional states. Taken voluntarily, most of these raise minimal ethical concerns, but the ethical concerns cannot be ignored either, given that almost all such compounds are addictive, and thus impair the ability of the person to grant or withhold voluntary consent to use them.

Brain enhancement through brain-machine interfaces, as mentioned in this book, are more challenging to evaluate ethically. For example, the use of brain signals performing internet searches etc., a form of 'mind-reading', could encroach on the fundamental right of humans to decide what information they choose to share with others. Technological progress in this regard may be inextricably tied to losses of privacy that the parties involved may eventually come to regret.

DR. KENNEDY'S RESEARCH JOURNEY

One of the most intriguing parts of this book is Phil's own story with the technology he invented. Like any other researcher who has come up with a new technique (in his case, the Neurotrophic Electrode), he started off focused on developing his technique as quickly as possible, to maximize its impact for helping patients and to propel his academic career. He learned along the way that academic success depends not only on the quality of one's research, but also on one's ability to generate adequate funding and to maneuver the regulatory landscape. Turning his patented technology (and others) into a commercial success was not an easy proposition, and FDA mandate restricted the number of patients in whom he was allowed to implant the device. This reflected the tension between the need to protect patients from unreasonable risks, and the need for data from patients to guide the further development of his technology so that it could help more patients.

He also learned that there were biological factors that limited his research. One is the fact that the patients who would most benefit from this technology often have multiple medical conditions, reducing their ability to fully participate in the research, and, of course, eventually to benefit from the use of this technology. Another is that the locked-in state of the patient impacts the amount of information that can be extracted from the experiments. As an example, it is highly important to the data analysis to know how the timing and extent of the patient's effort correlates to the electrical activity recorded from the brain. However, when a patient who cannot communicate is asked to 'say something in your mind', there is no way to know that the patient actually did so, and, if so, what the precise timing of the effort was. This 'ground truth' information is vital to Dr. Kennedy's work, as nuanced speech depends on rapid modulation of neuronal activities, and the electrical activity of individual neurons and ensembles of neurons is known to operate with millisecond precision. In many other fields of study, such considerations would lead researchers to conduct the research with healthy animals instead of severely ill humans. However, it is obviously not possible to study restoration of speech in subjects that are not able to speak in the first place. Alternatively, the problem could be addressed by conducting the research with either large groups of patients (so that common features revealed by group statistics are amplified over the variations among all the individuals), or in individuals who *can* communicate, in other words, healthy human beings. While the former is not feasible in this case because of resource limitations and regulatory restrictions, conducting such experiments on healthy research subjects is clearly ethically untenable.

As he details in this book, Phil eventually turned to the age-old solution of self-experimentation. Conducting experiments on his own brain would resolve many of the thorny issues that accompany the tests conducted on others. I imagine that Phil's hopes were very high when he first contemplated using himself as the research subject: He would not have to contend with the ethical issues that accompany device testing in others, some of the regulatory constraints would not apply, and, most importantly, he would have excellent control over some of the relevant experimental parameters.

Biological experimentation typically is most likely to lead to meaningful results if it adheres to a well-thought-out experimental plan, and if it pursues clear-cut testable hypotheses. On the other hand, 'exploratory' science, i.e., science done without pre-stated hypotheses, while generally not yielding scientific conclusions, may help to generate new hypotheses, or may help to hone technical methods. From an experimentalist's perspective the principal down-side of self-experimentation is that it provides data points from only a single subject, the researcher. As such, this type of research is (mostly) exploratory. Further, it is very difficult to control for bias in self-research. Biases in science have become a topic with ever-increasing importance in recent years. While biases are seldom conscious, even the best-intentioned researcher may not be able to avoid subtle adjustments to the experimental flow. It is feared that such adjustments or analysis tendencies may end up in outcomes that unduly support models the researcher may have. The recognition of this has led researchers to develop study designs that emphasize rigorous blinding of researchers, repetition of studies by independent investigators, collaborative studies (where different study sites provide checks and balances on one another) and the use of robust study designs where experiments are conducted to fulfill predetermined requirements of statistical power. Unfortunately, none of these are feasible with self-experiments like those done by Dr. Kennedy.

Self-experimentation carries other risks as well, including the risk of seriously affecting the health and well-being of the researcher who carries them out. In Phil's case, the implantation of the Neurotrophic Electrode(s) and associated hardware went well, but the postoperative period must have been a true test of his conviction of the need for this work, not to mention the devotion of his family. He found himself far from home, unable to speak (or write) for a few days after the operation, developed weakness, and had seizures. He knew that all of these were likely results of his brain swelling (and scarring?), related to the implantation and the presence of the Electrodes in his brain, but, at the time, he could not know when, or even whether, they would resolve. With appropriate medical treatment though, his speech returned, the seizures subsided, and he eventually returned to his home in the Atlanta area, where he proceeded to use the implanted Electrodes to examine the activity of his own brain. The period of experimentation was ultimately cut short when some of the hardware had to be removed because of other medical issues.

Phil made the most of the few weeks between the time when his brain had fully adapted to the presence of the Electrodes, and the medically necessitated removal of the hardware, taking advantage of the amazing fact that he was literally the only otherwise healthy person on the planet who could monitor actions of single nerve cells in his own brain. He used the time to study the relationship between his initiation of word fragments ('phones') and the activity of 'single units' recorded with his Electrodes (the term 'single unit' is used to refer to the firing activity of single nerve cells in the brain). While some of this work has been presented at scientific meetings and in publications like this book, much work remains to be done to complete the analysis. Most of the self-experimentation done by Dr.

Kennedy falls into the category of exploratory science (as defined above), and thus has to be followed up, preferably by other researchers, in other subjects, before the results can be accepted as scientific 'truths.' Nevertheless, the data have already given rise to improvements in the hardware and software approaches used for such work and may help to make future studies more accurate.

Overall, the risk-benefit calculation of this self-experiment would look unfavorable to many researchers, given the serious health effects Phil experienced. However, I'm sure that he disagrees. He likely would not think twice about repeating the experiment if he were to get a chance to do so.

MELODY MOORE JACKSON

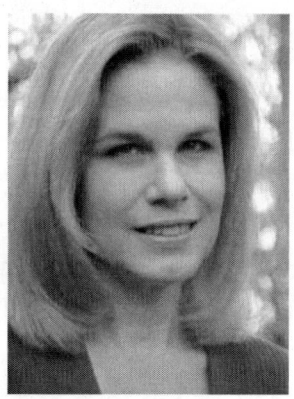

Dr. Jackson is the Director of the Georgia Tech BrainLab, whose mission is to research innovative human-computer interaction for people with severe disabilities, including direct brain interfaces and other biometric interfaces. She and her team have researched ways of improving communication, environmental control, mobility, and stroke rehabilitation with brain signal control. The BrainLab's current work also includes mobile DBI for mainstream users. Her work has been funded by the National Science Foundation, National Institutes of Health (NINDS), NIDRR, and DARPA.

Commentary

When we look at the contributions non-invasive techniques make to the locked-in person, over the last 22 years, beyond supporting Dr. Kennedy with his motor cortex implant research, my BrainLab team has also extensively studied non-surgical imaging methods to provide assistive technologies for people with severe disabilities. We have explored many aspects of EEG (electroencephalograph, measuring electrical activity in the brain), fNIR (functional near-infrared imaging), GSR (galvanic skin response, measuring changes in sweat on the skin, typically used for lie detection), and fMRI (functional Magnetic Resonance Imaging) that detects brain function, not just anatomy.

There are many different ways to use EEG to spell; the first we studied was motor imagery. The locked-in user would think about moving a hand or a foot, and we could detect the electrical activity in the brain to move a cursor on a virtual keyboard and "press" a selection button to choose a letter. We have also created keyboards that flash letters, and as the user focuses on the desired letter, we can see a brain response when that letter flashes (called P300, so named because this EEG signal reacts 300 ms after visualization of the desired letter). A third method is to flash letters or words at different frequencies - for example, flashing "yes" 15 times per second which distinguishes "yes" from "no" that is flashing 19 times per second - and looking for the corresponding frequency in the visual cortex, which means the user was focusing on that word. This technique is called SSVEP.

We have also implemented many other assistive technologies using EEG-based imaging. We created an environmental control system based on motor imagery that allowed the user to change the channel on the TV or radio, to turn the lights on and off, and to open and close the draperies in the home. We also created a communication system called "Health Talker" based on P300 that allowed a locked-in patient to point out areas of his or her body that had a problem, and then to describe what was wrong (pain, spasm, nausea, etc.).

We created two brain-driven wheelchairs; the "Aware Chair" used motor imagery to guide the chair, and also understood the context that the user was in. The 'chair' "knew" that it was time for the patient's favorite TV show and would give the user the option to automatically drive into the TV room, turn on the TV, and close the drapes, as well as texting a family member that the show was starting. The second wheelchair was based on SSVEP and was implemented by my student Michael Boyce (now Ph.D.), who reverse engineered his own power wheelchair to be brain-driven. He had a controller based on a grid of flashing checker boxes, and the chair would turn, go forward, or stop based on where Michael focused his gaze on the grid. We have also built robots based on EEG imaging; one of the robots made coffee with a P300-based control. The user would focus on flashing images of instant coffee, creamer, sugar, and stirring, and the robot could be directed to make coffee the way the user preferred. We have also created a brain-controlled drone with the same brain imaging method.

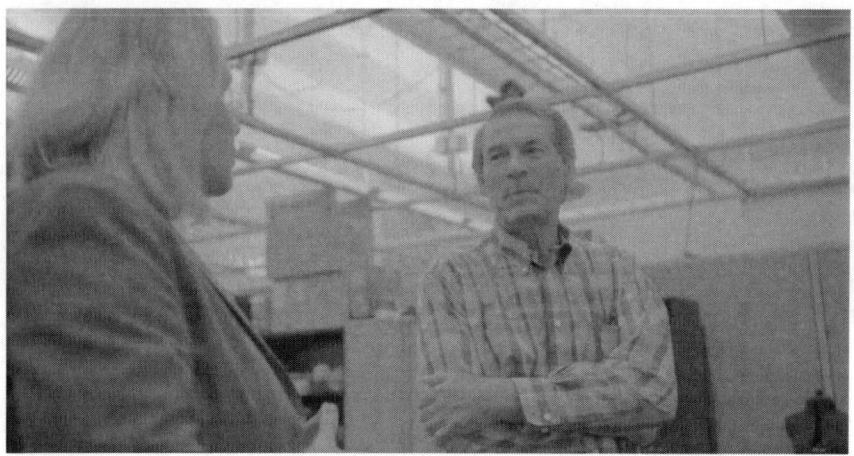

Professor Jackson talking with Dr. Kennedy. Screenshot from Documentary, "The Father of the Cyborgs."

The EEG systems are effective, but require a high level of expertise in applying the Electrodes to the scalp (often with a cap containing the Electrodes). The best imaging is obtained using a conductive gel, which is messy, and also dries out with extended use. So we have also studied two systems based on fNIR, which is simpler to set up, for communication instead. The first, built by a company called Archinoetics, was created for a locked-in artist in Hawaii. It allowed her to "paint" with her brain by using imagined language imagery (such as reciting a poem silently) to move a color wheel and a drawing cursor. Another system, the Kokoro-Gatari built by Hitachi, was designed for a late-stage ALS patient, and allowed the user to say "yes" or "no" based on language imagery. We performed one of the largest studies ever done with ALS patients at the time, bringing the machine to over 40 users all over the U.S. and collecting data for a span of two years.

Although it's not technically a brain-computer interface, we implemented a system based on galvanic skin response (GSR, better known as a police lie detector). A locked-in patient (NB) learned to use emotional imagery to raise his GSR on his fingers, which allowed him to select letters or phrases from a communication program.

We have also studied fMRI-based systems, and although it's not practical to require an MRI magnet to communicate, we can learn about brain activity and hopefully transfer these systems to a more portable imaging method such as EEG. Our BrainSign project used fMRI imaging on participants who knew American Sign Language (ASL) as they performed, and then simply imagined, sign language phrases. The method worked remarkably well, differentiating ten different sign language phrases with upwards of 90% accuracy from the brain activity alone. The advantage of a language, such as ASL, over spelling is that it is far more efficient. We are continuing studies like this with motor activation, seeking to create the fastest noninvasive brain-computer interface to date.

We are also currently working on EEG for auditory responses (ASSR) that allows the user to listen to pure tones, or even short speech bites, to make selections. These systems could provide a hands-free, eyes-free, voice-free control interface for emergency responders, drivers, astronauts, or anyone else whose attention needs to be focused on a primary task while still communicating. As part of this National Science Foundation funded study, we are also experimenting with ways of making brain-computer interfaces mobile, including creating in-ear Electrodes that can image brain signals with nothing more than an earbud for data recording.

182 Scientific Commentaries

At the other end of the spectrum, when we ask where we are with non-invasive technologies and conversational speech, the challenge for any brain-computer interface is the speed of communication. Even the fastest spelling systems top out at about 8 characters per minute. Therefore, solutions such as using American Sign Language, which represents words rather than letters, makes conversation more feasible. But currently brain-computer interface communication systems are slow relative to the 120-150 words per minute of natural speech.

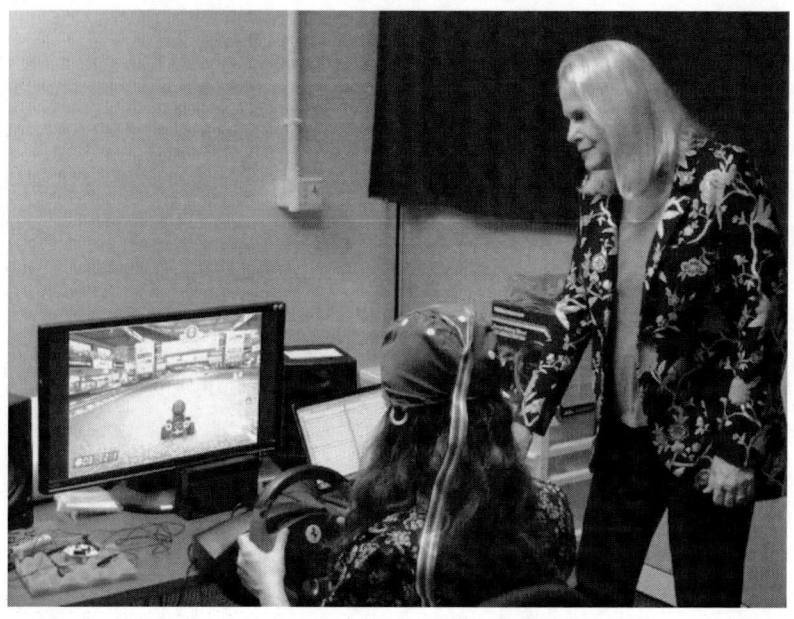

In a simpler setting, like trying for accurate finger movements with non-invasive techniques, it is possible to control movement (such as finger movement, or navigating a wheelchair) *smoothly and accurately* if more of the "smarts" is in the device. For example, our coffee-making robot was programmed to perform the steps of making coffee - dip the spoon into the instant coffee, move to the coffee cup, turn the spoon over. All of those movements were one selection from the brain-computer interface. Finer control, which might be required for more arbitrary tasks such as feeding oneself a grape, would be very difficult with non-invasive techniques.

However, John Donoghue's BrainGate (an *invasive* system) did allow a patient to perform that exact task accurately.

Of course, the big question is, can today's research produce sufficient data to provide conversational speech? As with smooth finger movement, the more "smarts" we can put in the device, the better the conversation. There are word-completion and sentence-completion programs that can help predict things that the user might say to speed up augmented communication. Our "Aware Chair" project included a predictive conversation generator that altered the phrases available for user selection based on time of day, place (work, home, hospital), people in the room (your mother, your friend, your doctor) and conversational history with the people in the room. Therefore, in the morning, the phrase "good evening" would not be present. If the user's friend loves basketball, the system would go to the internet and pull up the latest basketball news in the presence of that friend, and provide conversational suggestions such as "hey, did you see the Hawks beat the Lakers?". If the user was at the doctor, it would provide appropriate medical questions and symptom reports. However, it is unlikely that something as flexible as phones will be possible to detect noninvasively, in contrast to what Dr. Kennedy's lab has been working on.

One large growth area across the whole BCI field is how AI (neural net paradigms) enhance the decoding of data streams. AI, specifically machine learning, is critical to the classifiers that we use to decode brain signals. Machine learning systems look for patterns in data, and try to categorize those patterns so we can attach meaning to them. Neural nets are just one method of pattern matching paradigms, but there are many others (Hidden Markov Models, Principal Component Analysis, Linear Discriminant Analysis, to name just a few we have experimented with). Our BrainLab team includes several machine learning researchers who are constantly working to refine and improve our classifier methods.

But setting aside the technology competencies for a moment, I really would like to describe what it was like, working with our incredible "test pilot" patients, who all deserve sainthood. Here are a few of my favorite stories about these inspiring men.

JR

I joined Dr. Kennedy's team very shortly after JR's implant surgery so I was privileged to be there for his initial training. JR was a delightful, sweet man with a keen sense of humor, and even though he was completely locked-in from a brainstem stroke, he could still smile with his eyes and move a few muscles on his face. We worked with him nearly every day for four years, and he was one of the strongest and toughest men I have ever met. He tested everything we came up with, and even helped us improve our systems with his own suggestions. He showed us his sense of humor when we created a virtual hand for him, which was controlled by the implanted Electrode. He imagined moving his own fingers, and the virtual fingers would move. We were chagrined when the first thing he did was move just one of the fingers - the middle one, sticking it up in a questionable gesture. He clearly thought that was hilarious and we all laughed and laughed. JR was definitely a character.

But the most poignant moment with JR was during one of our sessions when he was using a speller, about two years into the project. We discovered that the motor imagery that JR used to move the cursor on the screen would change - sometimes day to day. We would ask him, "what are you thinking about to move the cursor today?" and he would spell "foot", or "hand", or "tongue".

But on that day, he spelled "nothing". Dr. Kennedy and I looked at each other in puzzlement. "Nothing?" we said. Then JR spelled, "thinking of moving the cursor". The enormity of that simple phrase hit us, and we had to go out into the hall to catch our breath. JR's brain had assimilated the task of moving the cursor, and he no longer had to use motor imagery. He just "willed" the cursor to move, and it did. We certainly knew that neuroplastic change is a possibility in the brain, but to see it illustrated so clearly and dramatically was a highlight of my career.

Scientific Commentaries 185

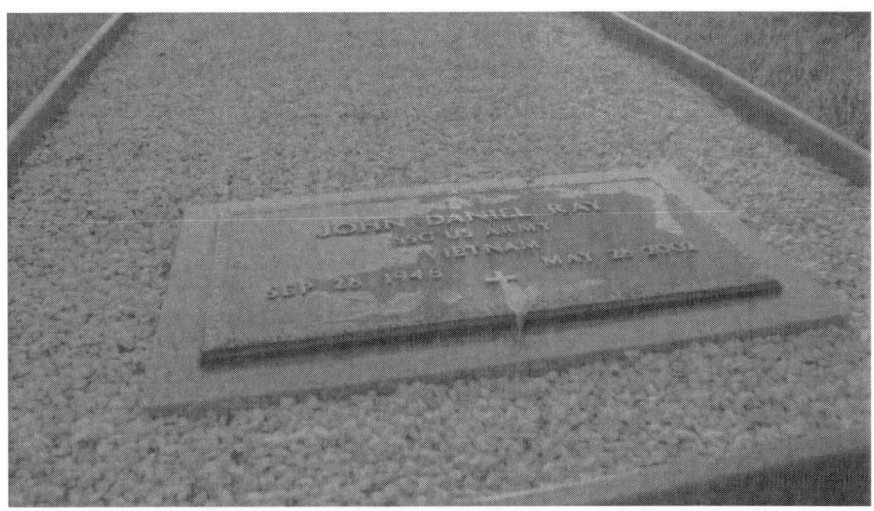

The grave site of JR, the world's first cyborg. Screenshot from Documentary, "The Father of the Cyborgs."

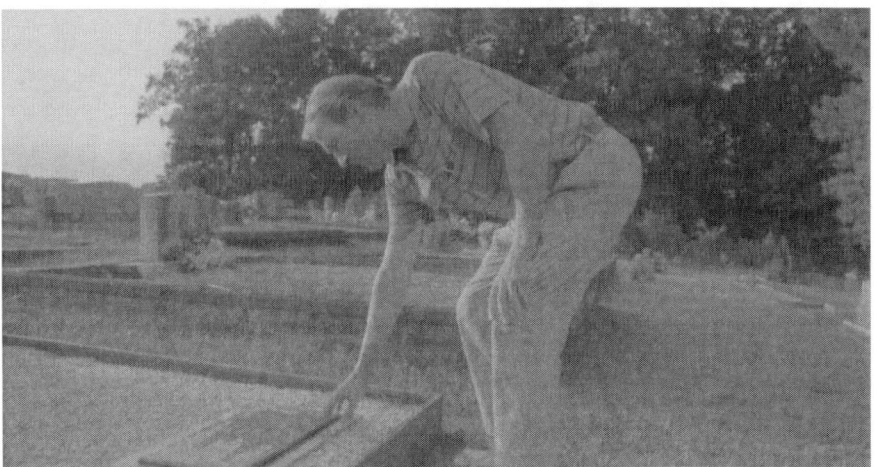

At the grave site of JR, the world's first cyborg. Dr. Kennedy visits his grave every year at the Sandy Flat's gravesite just outside Bowdon, Georgia. Screenshot from Documentary, "The Father of the Cyborgs."

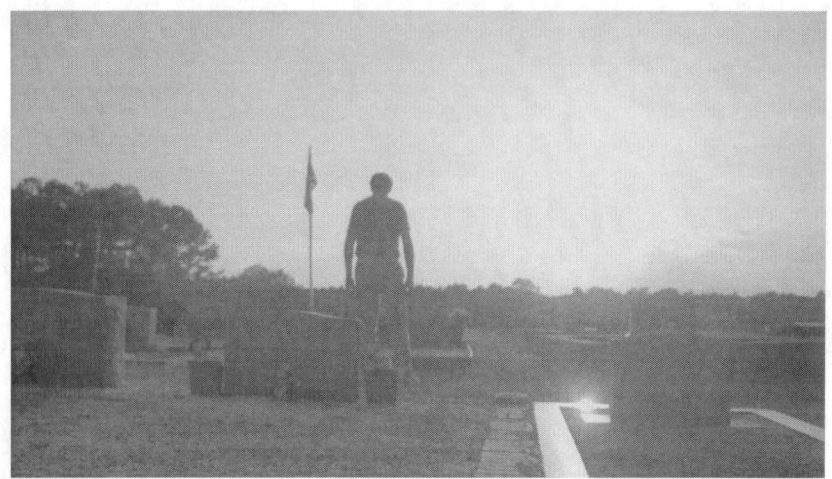

At the grave site of JR, the world's first cyborg. Screenshot from Documentary, "The Father of the Cyborgs."

TT

TT was the second implant patient that I was able to work with; he was completely locked-in from a rare progressive mitochondrial myopathy. He was a younger man, who had been a bit of a rebel, and a picture of him on his motorcycle was always at his bedside. When he first came to Atlanta he could move his eyes only slightly, but that allowed him a way to say yes and no, and to move his eyes to "point" at letters or phrases in a book that he brought with him. I spent hours and hours learning to communicate with him, and we had many meaningful conversations. When he went in for his surgery he asked me with tears in his eyes if I was going to be there. I assured him I was, and asked him if he was afraid. He said, "no. But can't talk". He wanted to make sure his "interpreter" was close by. And of course I was there, and glad to do it.

TT did many of the things that JR did, spelling with the virtual keyboard. He was never as successful as JR, probably because he had been locked-in for years rather than months as JR had been, and the mitochondrial disease affected his brain cells as well as his muscles. So we tried other methods, such as P300 which only requires attention to flashing stimuli. The most important system we created for him was Health Talker, which came about from a frustrating but illuminating situation. As with JR, we visited TT every day. The first thing we would ask him was "do you have any pain?" and if he said yes, we would play 20 questions to figure out what was hurting. "Is it your feet?" "Is it your stomach?" "Is it your head?", and then we would go through the list of things that could be wrong with that body part. TT had fairly frequent spasms, and he could end up with his feet painfully crossed or sores on his head. So one day we began our visit with the usual questions. "Do you have any pain?" "yes". "Is it your feet?" "no". I went through the entire list of things that could be wrong, and finally, "Is it your stomach?" "YES". OK, now we were getting somewhere. "Are you nauseated?" "no". "Does your stomach hurt?" "no". hmmm. After asking everything I could think of about his stomach, all of the answers were "no". TT was becoming more agitated and frustrated, but I was determined to figure it out. Finally, I asked, "do you mind if I lift the sheet and check your stomach?" and he agreed. When I lifted the sheet, I saw that he was lying in a puddle of tan-colored liquid. I realized then that his feeding tube had come out of his stomach, and the liquid food was just being pumped onto his skin. Who knows how long he had been lying in his breakfast, but it certainly couldn't have been comfortable. After notifying his medical staff, we started designing the HealthTalker system that would allow him to choose a body part, and then a description of what might be wrong, using a P300 selection mechanism. We never again wanted to have to play the 20-questions game for him to tell us something was wrong like that.

DJ

DJ was a larger-than life character, a successful young stockbroker and avid outdoorsman, who was struck by ALS while still in his twenties and over the years became completely locked-in except for a small hand movement and muscles on his face. He lived a very long time with his ALS, close to 30 years, and he was a primary test pilot for many of our studies in the nearly 20 years that I worked with him. DJ was an implant patient, but complications from the surgery required the implant to be removed. However, we continued to work with him on a regular basis with noninvasive projects for years, and he was a huge contributor to our research. He eventually lost control of his hand muscles, but continued to be able to drive his wheelchair and spell fairly quickly with a word-prediction program and a cheek switch mounted to a pair of glasses. DJ even traveled to Georgia Tech to do a talk with me about our research... crafting his presentation and presenting it via voice synthesizer. He also had been a prolific fisherman and hunter, and during one of our visits, he proudly pointed out a new stuffed bobcat on his mantel. I asked when he had bagged it, and he said "3 months ago." I'm sure my jaw dropped, because I had been working with him about 10 years at that point; I had assumed he had shot it when he was still able-bodied. He proceeded to describe a system that a friend had rigged on his wheelchair, that allowed him to aim a crossbow by moving the wheelchair up and down, and then firing the crossbow with his cheek switch. He hit the bobcat, perfectly, from 50 yards, with his assistive system. Needless to say, we were all floored (and wishing we had thought of building that!)

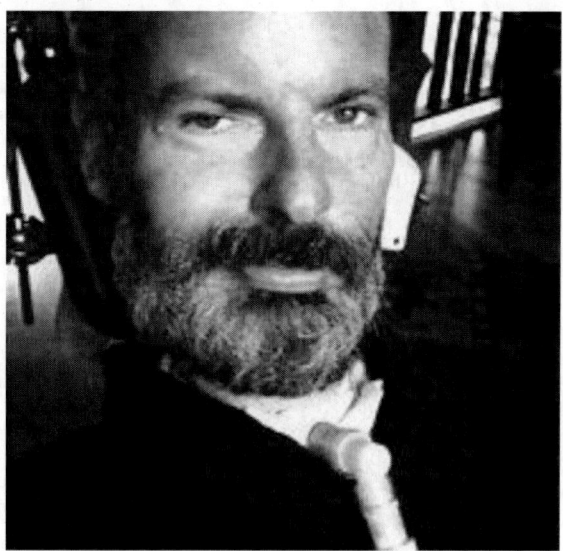

DJ tested just about everything we created, from the fNIR communication system, to the P300 speller, to the SSVEP-based environmental control system. About two years ago he contracted skin cancer (no doubt from many hours in the sun) and had extensive surgery on his face. He also had pneumonia several times through the years. He struggled with recovery from his cancer surgery and the constant financial difficulties that being locked-in caused. Last summer (June 13, 2018), he opted to turn off his ventilator. I sat with him the night before, with his friends and family gathered around, celebrating his extraordinary contribution to this world. I gave him a Georgia Tech cap (he was a rabid Georgia fan, long-term rivals, so he grimaced), but told him it was because he was the center of the BrainLab. The GT BrainLab is named for him now, and I will never forget this courageous, caring, funny, smart man who was such an integral part of our research team.

NB

NB was also an extraordinary man; he was a brilliant eye surgeon who had been a pioneer in the Lasik technique and then contracted ALS in his forties. He lived with his parents in Beverly Hills, and the family even built a guest house for our team to stay in when we visited. He initially considered having the Kennedy implant, but he had some- mitigating factors and decided not to try it. However, we continued to work with him with noninvasive techniques for many years until he succumbed to his ALS. NB tested our first fNIR system along with many of the EEG based spelling systems, as well as our GSR-based system. He had around-the-clock nursing care, because he couldn't blink his eyes, and therefore needed to have eye drops added every few minutes. During one visit, we noticed that NB was a bit agitated as we set up the system for that day's training session. He seemed eager for us to get his communication system hooked up, so we hurried. The first thing he did was spell "Annie fired". His mother, who was in the room, gasped. "Why?" she asked. "Sleep", he spelled. Apparently Annie was his night nurse, who instead of taking care of him and putting the drops in his eyes, was sleeping through the night. She assumed that he was a vegetable and that he couldn't rat her out, but she was sorely mistaken. The fact that NB could have that measure of control over his life - he fired her himself using our spelling system - was one of the most triumphant achievements of our work. The look of shock on her face is something I'll never forget, and the satisfaction from his wonderful family that he could tell them about his quality of care was priceless.

NICK RAMSEY

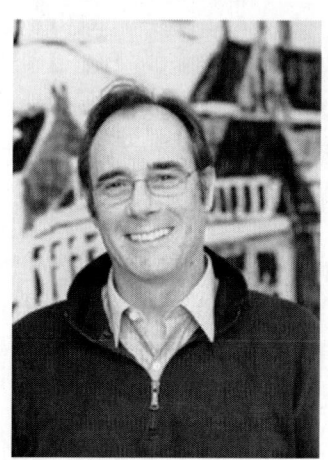

Nick Ramsey has a degree in Psychology and a PhD in neuropsychopharmacology, both from the university of Utrecht (Netherlands). He became a specialist in cognitive neuroimaging in the US (National Institutes of Health, 1995), and applies modern techniques, including fMRI and intracranial EEG, to questions on working memory, language, and sensorimotor function. His goal is to acquire and translate neuro-scientific insights to patients with brain disorders, with a focus on brain-computer interfacing (BCI). He is professor in cognitive neuroscience at the University Medical Center of Utrecht since 2007. The research on BCI since 2005 resulted in the first case of home use of a fully implanted intracranial EEG BCI implant in a Locked-in patient (NEJM 2016, Clin Neurophysiol 2019). His current research aims to restore speech in severely paralyzed people. In 2015 he founded spin-off company Braincarta that offers clinically validated functional MRI mapping for neurosurgery.

Commentary

I met Phil almost 15 years ago, at the annual Society for Neuroscience conference where we talked about his work with Erik. I learned about his Neurotrophic Electrodes too, and was fascinated. The way it was fabricated made a lot of sense for long-term use. Since then we've run into each other pretty much every year, always talking about Erik and later Phil's own implant. When we first met, only a few people had been implanted with a BCI, most of them participating in Phil's research. But others were starting to implant too, as was my lab in the Netherlands. And somehow Phil's program lost steam despite the promising technology he used. How come? There are several potential reasons I can think of, perhaps the most important of which is not being able to get new FDA approval for investigational use of the technology. Over the years the rules for human implants have become more strict, including more safeguards in the process. Writing a protocol to get approval today requires a team of scientists and a lot of time. It also requires patience and a willingness to think in regulatory terms as well as considerable funding and a much higher cost of making the device. All in all a lot of writing instead of doing the hard research.

Phil may not be the person to follow that path. He conducted the research with one patient at a time and different approaches to discover what works. He was an early explorer. Phil also was the first to implant the amplifiers, avoiding wires running through the skin. Implanting electronics increases the scrutiny by FDA for patient safety, adding to the regulatory burden for Phil to continue his work. As Phil describes in this book, implantation of experimental devices can lead to medical problems. The modern day high standards for medical device design and production intend to reduce such risks. I considered using Phil's system in our patients, but we quickly found out that approval for experimental use would require a complete redesign of the system to meet safety requirements. So, with FDA approval missing, what to think of Phil implanting himself? In modern science this is frowned upon, especially if it involves a device that is not approved. Nobody else would then be able to immediately benefit from the findings. Yet, it certainly demonstrates Phil's faith in his technology and his dedication to the science.

And to be fair, had medical problems not forced Phil to have his device removed, we could have learned much more about the neural signals for communication. Having said that though, some of the research on that can now be conducted with electrocorticography, where experiments can be performed with patients who have Electrodes placed over the brain to identify the source of seizures. Between the medical diagnostic procedures, brain signals can be investigated for communication from the same area that Phil has been investigating. Regarding the Neurotrophic Electrodes, however, no other research exists to further develop the technology, in spite of the clear advantage that the signals last for many more years than the Electrodes that are currently used to record from single cells.

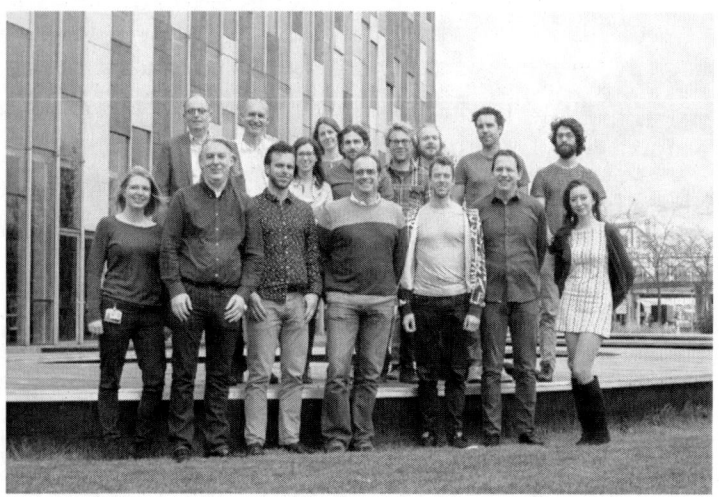

The story of Erik Ramsey is unique. Ten years of participation in research is impressive and shows a mutual commitment. Throughout the book the reader gets ample insight into life in locked-in state and the multitude of difficulties encountered in care at all levels. Phil also succeeds in translating the complex jargon of BCI research to understandable language. The book is pleasant to read, and provides information that cannot be found in the scientific articles Phil published. Phil's story, along with Erik Ramsey's story, is one of adventure and excitement. It is also a story with a beginning and an end. Without a doubt, Phil contributed to the now evolving field of BCI implants, and to the rising awareness of what it means to be locked-in.

BCI implants here at the Ramsey lab utilize Electrodes that lay on the surface of the brain with each Electrode recording electrical activity of several hundred-thousand neurons. Neural populations of this size, also called neuronal ensembles, exhibit very specific functions, such as moving a single finger or hearing a particular tone. When a paralyzed person wants to move a finger, actual movement does not occur but the neural activity does, and can be detected with these 'electrocorticography' (ECoG) Electrodes. Our Ramsey team has successfully used implanted ECoG Electrodes to enable a completely paralyzed person to communicate via a computer, doing so by turning brain signals into clicks that navigate a cursor through menus and an on-screen keyboard. The system has proved to be so reliable that the user has come to depend on the system for daily interactions with caregivers at home! With more capable hardware, the Ramsey team hopes to be able to eventually translate internal speech to a computer-generated voice, thus able to restore communication in those people with speech disabilities.

AYSEGUL GUNDUZ

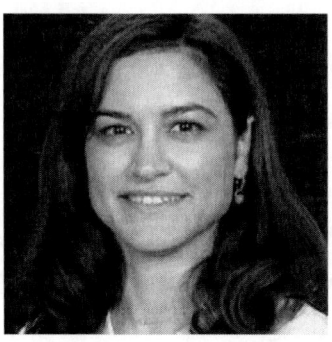

Dr. Aysegul Gunduz is an Associate Professor and University of Florida Research Foundation Professor at the J. Crayton Pruitt Family Department of Biomedical Engineering at the University of Florida. Her research interests include neural interfacing, neural signal processing, and neuromodulation in human subjects. She works with many neurosurgical patient populations such as patients suffering from essential tremor, Parkinson's disease, Tourette syndrome, and epilepsy. Her lab studies both motor and cognitive symptoms of these disorders and aims to develop novel therapies. Dr. Gunduz earned her BS, MS, and PhD degrees in Electrical Engineering from Middle East Technical University (Ankara, Turkey, 2001), North Carolina State University (Raleigh, NC, 2003), and University of Florida (Gainesville, FL, 2008), respectively. She received postdoctoral training at Albany Medical College, Department of Neurology, and at the Wadsworth Center, Division of Translational Medicine in Albany, NY. Dr. Gunduz is the recipient of the Presidential Early Career Award for Scientists and Engineers (PECASE, 2019), which is the highest honor bestowed by the U.S. government on outstanding scientists and engineers beginning their independent careers. Her other national and international honors include the National Science Foundation Early CAREER Award (2016), International Academy of Medical and Biological Engineering Early Career Award (2015), and Anita Borg Institute for Women in Technology Denice Denton Emerging Leader ABIE Award (2017).

Commentary

Today, I enjoy the fact that neural interfacing is a field that can excite the general public. Even a three-minute elevator pitch in our scientific area is easy and fun, and almost anyone will start up a conversation with me typically involving a loved one who is affected by a neurological disorder—whether it be Parkinson's disease, epilepsy, or ALS. People like interacting with brain scientists as they want to learn more about this mysterious organ, which can cause so much loss to the quality of life to the sufferer as well as their families, what Dr. Kennedy calls the "here and now". I enjoy reading popular books in this field, just like the general public, and I get inspired by them.

These books are now helping us overcome some myths about the brain, such as "we only use 10 percent of our brains," or classifying people as "left- or right-brained" (with gray colored left hemispheres to represent logic and right hemispheres bursting in color to represent artistry!).

As scientists in the field, it is our responsibility to demystify neural interfacing or brain-computer interfaces and provide public outreach. While I dislike users of neural interfaces being called "cyborgs," as I think in popular culture cyborgs are associated with humanoids that have destructive powers, generally I do understand the term has several meanings. Words or terms like *cyborgs*, *enhancement*, *mind-control* tend to make people nervous and can be detrimental to the field.

Let's just say that, first and foremost, we need to translate neuroscientific advances and discoveries so others can see that they improve the quality of life of those with neurological disorders. The field of neuro ethics is rapidly growing along with neural interfacing, and will hopefully keep associated terms and claims more down to earth.

When we think about whether an invasive neural interface is ethical to implant in a human, we must consider its risk-to-benefit ratio. For someone like Erik, who is locked-in, the benefits would be life-changing. But we still cannot ignore the risks. Regulatory agencies, such as the Food & Drug Administration (FDA) in the US, who also want to minimize this ratio, have to track preclinical trials closely.

I believe readers might be interested in this book since they may read about Dr. Phil Kennedy's story of voluntarily undergoing implantation of the Neurotrophic Electrodes. He developed this specialized Electrode himself and had FDA approval since 1998. His study lost FDA approval due to lack of unobtainable information about the trophic factors placed inside the Electrode tip.

Let me say as a young doctoral engineering student entering the field of brain-computer interfaces in 2004, I never thought *I* would have a chance to meet Dr. Kennedy in person, who is a pioneer in this field—let alone be one of the initial experts to have the privilege of reading parts of this book prior to publication.

Many of us today show proof-of-concept of brain-computer interfaces in patients that receive Electrode implants as part of their therapy independent of a need for such communication channels (e.g., epilepsy patients undergoing resective surgery, who are not locked in). Dr. Kennedy's work was unique when I joined the field, because he started his work with patients who would directly benefit from the technology. I think neuroethicists will discuss his decisions and self-implantation for years to come.

The "for" arguments will include the fact that he provided informed consent and that he did it for the benefit of science. The "against" arguments will repeatedly underline the huge risks for a healthy person to undergo brain surgery without clinical indication, but with a clear research imperative. The data from his recordings demonstrate that silent speech can be decoded off line, as described briefly in the book. Only time will reveal further benefits of the data that was collected from him and his early subjects. We will continue to benefit from the results.

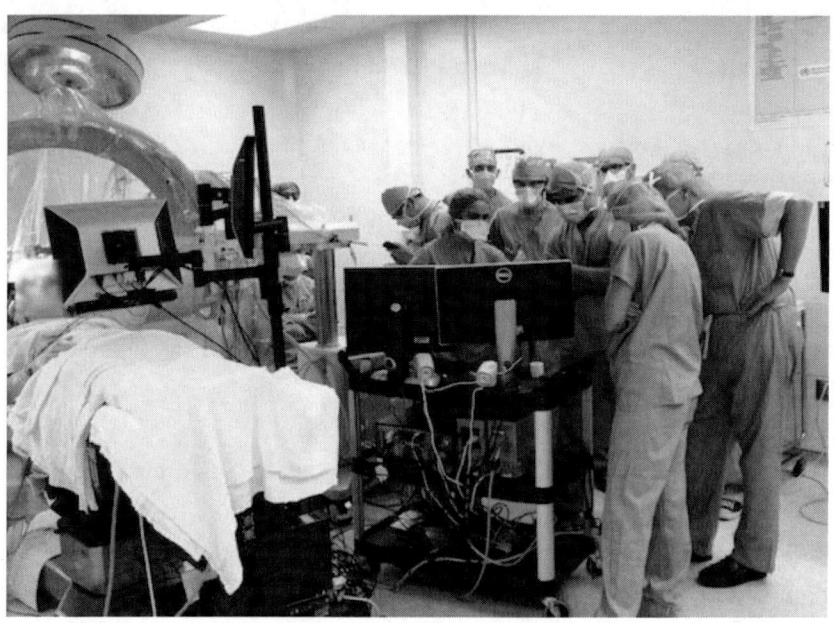

Dr. Gunduz is in the center of the photograph instructing the surgical team.

Afterword

The Father of the Cyborgs by David Burke

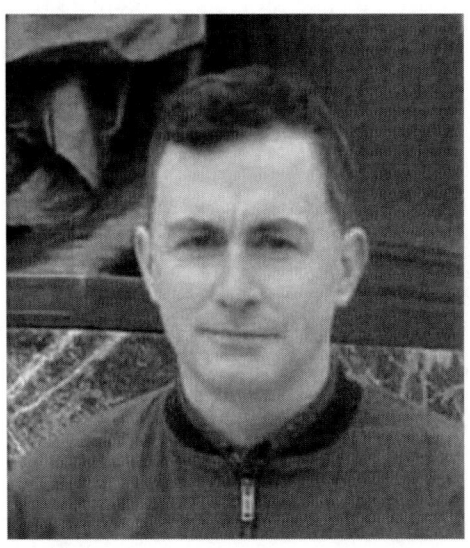

David Burke is an award-winning Irish documentary filmmaker. His first documentary *Men of the Rás* in 2012 was the Critics Choice in *The Irish Times* where it was described as a "gem." It won both the Best Sport and Overall Prize at the 2013 Celtic Media Festival. His second film, the feature documentary *Crash and Burn,* screened at numerous festivals nationally and internationally, receiving universal 4 star reviews in publications such as *The Irish Times* and *The Guardian*. It had a theatrical release and was subsequently broadcast on RTE in Ireland and the BBC in the U.K. It won Best Sports documentary at both the 2017 Celtic Media Festival and the 2018 Irish Film Television Awards.

During the filming of *The Father Of The Cyborgs* Phil mentioned the role serendipity plays in his research. He believes it's best to approach research with an open mind rather than looking for a specific outcome. It's what Nobel Prize winning scientist Paul Nurse refers to as 'getting off the tracks,' Nurse believes when you have an expected outcome it becomes increasing difficult to think of alternative answers and ideas, thus the analogy of the railway tracks.

The fact that some, or indeed many, of the best ideas are as a result of serendipity should bring to attention the state of mind, which seems to yield the best results. As a documentary film maker I believe if you keep your 'ear close to the ground 'an idea of interest will always make itself known, after all, given the time it takes to raise finance and shoot a documentary, you really only need one good idea a year! But therein lies the rub!

In order to be good at anything, it requires practice; this relates to spotting good ideas in the same way an expert art dealer can spot future trends or indeed the same way the experienced scientist is attracted to a piece of data which holds the key to a new breakthrough.

This brings me to another thing Phil mentioned: information is different to knowledge. In order to find one good idea it takes constant vigilance and a sifting process. In documentaries the road to one good idea is through 1000 bad ones. The two previous documentaries I produced came as a result of this process: a quixotic blend of vigilance, practice, serendipity and most definitely blind luck.

When it came to *The Father Of The Cyborgs* I did something different: I consciously went looking for an idea in the bio-engineering field. While the area itself is fascinating, I was at the time motivated to find out more about the kind of people who would be attracted to this field. A lot of searching led me to a short article about a neuroscientist who had implanted his own brain! Coming from a position of ignorance, my mind immediately jumped to the macabre and a firestorm of questions: where could one go to have your brain implanted? Did he enhance his brain? What was he hoping to achieve? Was I curious to know more: hell yes!

As I delved further into this field the material became stronger, richer, bolder and dare I say, madder. Everything from the history of brain implants, with characters/scientists like Jose Delgado and William Galbraith Heath to the timeliness of the subject matter with Facebook and Elon Musk announcing their current projects, was thoroughly compelling. Paul Nurse's tracks had not just been ripped up but molded into a new world that was challenging the very nature of what it meant to be human. Even taking this into account, the piece of information that surprised me the most was that Phil Kennedy was from Limerick! Twenty miles from where I was seated at the time. I had to try reach out to him.

Fortunately Phil was coming to Ireland around this time and on the way to our first meeting, my overriding thoughts were: I better 'bring my A-Game' as I waited for the pioneering neuroscientist! Phil as I have later learned, doesn't really "do" needless stress and was very open to my ideas on a documentary about his life work.

It was decided the best approach was to look for development funding from the Irish Film agency, Screen Ireland, and so we received seed funding to make a short teaser clip, and then on to attract further funding to make the documentary proper.

It was during the production of this teaser clip we met Phil's past patient David Jayne, and the father of Erik, Eddie Ramsey, a major strand of the documentary became immediately apparent. Their strength of character in the face of seemingly insurmountable odds was awe inspiring. In the presence of these real life pioneers, the Elon Musks and Facebooks of the world cannot compete with the best elements of just being human.

While the documentary would of course discuss the far-reaching possibilities of Brain-Computer Interfacing, the most important element was the human one.

When discussing Phil's self-experimentation, ethicist Paul Root Wolpe of Emory University referred to it as an 'interesting tension' inherent in this kind of work and, at least in this case, a brain better knowing itself, we might say. I also felt that this phrase could be applied to the wider advancement of Brain-Computer Interfacing. It is this "interesting tension" that is ubiquitous throughout the film and isn't confined to the ethics of self-experimentation. The film examines the dichotomy between the original intention for this technology, to help people with disabilities, with the unintended consequences it could have, as human brains get closer to a symbiosis with technology. I knew the documentary had to deftly balance the possible tech driven future with the altruistic possibilities this technology holds. It is this tension that is at the heart of the film, and informs the book.

Timing can be a key element across all areas of life and with neurotechnology such a hot topic at the moment in Silicon Valley is an example where there has been a surge of interest in Brain Computer Interfacing (BCI). For example, with Bryan Johnson, Facebook and Elon Musk among others, investing heavily in this technology, with both medical and consumer motivations. Musk has stated that his goal is to merge the human brain with AI. With Phil widely regarded as one of the pioneers of this technology, he is uniquely placed to discuss the far reaching consequences and ramifications of BCI, and this certainly helped attract the funding we needed to begin production of the documentary that tracks early breakthroughs in the field.

Thinking about the abstract nature of thought and our brain's relationship with our environment offered up a number of opportunities visually to tell this story in an original and compelling way. Aerial footage of the environment Phil occupies throughout the film will act as a subtle metaphor for the brain itself. As he opens the film describing the brain as a series of waves; spectacular footage of the Co. Kerry coast act as a visual metaphor for the brain. Similarly, cityscapes will be used to describe the brain immersed in modern technology as well as acting as introductory shots to particular sequences.

One of the first scenes I envisaged for the documentary was following Phil on his annual visit to the grave of his patient JR, to the Baptist Church in Bowdon, on the Georgia/Alabama State Line. It terms of imagery, I felt this could be an interesting way of introducing this sequence into the documentary. Some commentators have also alluded to the religious overtones in some of the ideas expressed in modern science: once people sought immorality through salvation from God and now some are seeking immortality through science. It also had the human element mentioned previously; a doctor paying homage to a former patient, whom he respected greatly.

At the grave of the 'World's First Cyborg' these worlds would meet in a way I hadn't envisioned. The Pastor from the Church, didn't just want to welcome us to his Church, he was intent on saving our souls! With heads bowed, for 20 minutes in the carpark, he asked us to look deep into our souls and to invite Jesus in. One of the crew remarked to me afterwards he looked up at one point to see Phil looking at the pastor with a bemused look on his face! The pastor later posted on social media a picture of 'the 5 souls from Ireland who were saved in the carpark of Bowdon Baptist Church' so who am I to disagree!

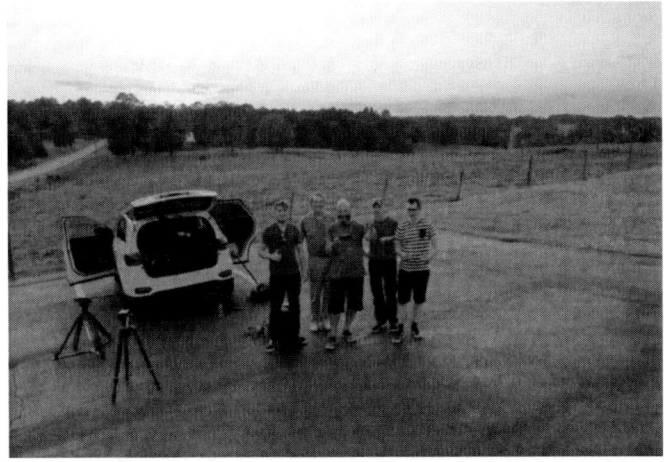

The five saved souls from Ireland are from left, Keith Pendred; Camera Operator, Phil Kennedy, JJ Rolfe; Director of Photography, Alan Poole; Sound Operator and myself Director/Producer.

When we returned from our first shoot in Atlanta I sent a brief email thanking Eddie Ramsey for his time and received a remarkable reply; in it Eddie had a suggestion to help us fully appreciate what being locked-in is like. In order to fully understand Erik's condition, he described how he lay motionless for up to 2 -3 days on separate occasions so he could have a greater appreciation of what his son was going through!

I was delighted to learn that Phil was producing the book *Unlocking Erik* with writer Brian Shaw. Together Phil, Erik and Eddie created the world's first speech BCI. Remarkably Facebook is now promoting the same proof of concept to develop their 'silent speech' BCI for the consumer market. For me however, there is something far more important to this story and why it deserves to be explored in depth. Phil's motivation for developing this technology is to help patients, not to profit from it financially. Eddie personifies to me many of the best human traits, although I'm sure he'll be embarrassed by me saying this! He gave half his life in sole pursuit of helping his son.

Phil describes many of his patients as heroes, and, in fact, they made great personal sacrifices knowing that the benefits reaped will be for future generations. If, or indeed when, BCI does become ubiquitous, the people pushing this technology forward will need to share many of these qualities. Endeavours pursued solely for profits inevitably create more social problems than they fix.

Our ethics and morals of today may very well shape who we become tomorrow. By reading *Unlocking Erik*, and in viewing *The Father of Cyborgs* you can take an unforgettable journey into the heart of what it really means to be human.

In Memory of Roy Bakay, MD by Phil Kennedy This research could not have been successful without the enthusiasm and surgical skills of Roy. Here we are on our first visit to Belize in 2013.

He decided he would be an oral surgeon and I would be an ENT surgeon! Graduation picture is below. His sense of humor helped us through some tough times! He is sorely missed. His support was always powerful and essential.

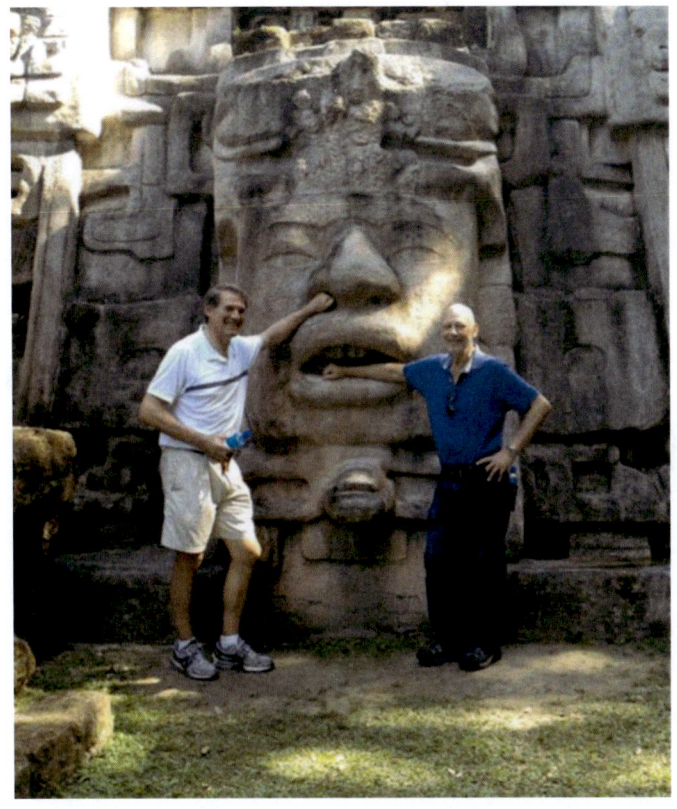

REFERENCES

To examine the data in greater depth, go to www.nlm.nih.gov, click on PubMed and enter the reference. For some references a short summary is provided in footnotes.

[1] Kennedy, P. R. (1989) A long-term Electrode that records from neurites grown onto its recording surface. *J. Neuroscience Methods*, 29: 181-193.

[2] Kennedy, P. R., Andreasen, D. S., Bartels, J., Ehirim,P., Wright, E. J., Seibert, S. and Cervantes, A. J. Validation of Neurotrophic Electrode long-term recordings in human cortex. *Handbook of Biomedical Engineering*. 2018.

[3] Homer M. L., Nurmikko A. V., Donoghue J. P. and Hochberg L. R. Sensors and decoding for intracortical brain computer interfaces *Annual Rev Biomed Eng.* 2013;15:383-405.

[4] Kennedy P. R. and Bakay R. A. E. Restoration of neural output from a paralyzed patient by a direct brain connection. *Neuroreport.* 1998 Jun 1;9(8):1707-11.

[5] Kennedy, P. R., Bakay, R. A. E., Adams, K., Goldthwaite, J. and Moore, M. Direct control of a computer from the human central nervous system. *IEEE Trans. Rehab. Eng.,* 8(2), 198-202, 2000.

[6] Kennedy, P. R. and King, B. Dynamic interplay of neural signals during the emergence of cursor related cursor in a human implanted with the Neurotrophic Electrode. CH 7 in *Neural Prostheses for Restoration of Sensory and Motor Function.* Eds. Chapin, J. and Moxon, K. CRC Press, 2001.

[7] Kennedy, P. R., Mirra, S. and Bakay, R. A. E. The Cone Electrode: Ultrastructural Studies Following Long-Term Recording. *Neuroscience Letters,* 142:89-94, (1992).

[8] Fetz, E. E. and Baker, M,A. Operantly conditioned patterns on precentral unit activity and correlated responses in adjacent cells and contralateral muscles. *J Neurophysiol.* 1973 Mar;36(2):179-204.

[9] Cheetah software called Cluster Cutting from Neuralynx Inc. of Boise, Montana, USA (www.neuralynx.com).

[10] LDA is linear discriminant analysis, SVM is support vector machine and FDA is Functional Data Analysis. For further explanation consult a statistical analysis source.

[11] Kennedy, P. R. Changes in emotional state modulate neuronal firing rates in human speech motor cortex: A case study in long-term recording. *Neurocase,* (2011) 17(5): 381-393

[12] MATLAB. The MathWorks, Inc., 3 Apple Hill Drive, Natick, MA 01760-2098.

[13] Downey, J. E., Schwed, N., Chase, S. M., Schwartz, A. B. and Collinger, J. L. Intracortical recording stability in human brain-computer interface users. *J Neural Eng.* 2018 Aug;15(4):046016.

[14] Collinger, J. L., Wodlinger, B., Downey, J. E., Wang, W., Tyler-Kabara, E. C., Weber, D. J., McMorland, A. J., Velliste, M., Boninger, M. L. and Schwartz, A. B. High-performance neuroprosthetic control by an individual with tetraplegia. *Lancet.* 2013 Feb 16;381(9866):557-64.

[15] Ajiboye, A. B., Willett, F. R., Young, D. R., Memberg, W. D., Murphy, B. A., Miller, J. P., Walter, B. L., Sweet, J. A., Hoyen, H. A., Keith, M. W., Peckham, P. H., Simeral, J. D., Donoghue, J. P., Hochberg, L. R. and Kirsch, R.F. Restoration of reaching and grasping movements through brain-controlled muscle stimulation in a person

with tetraplegia: a proof-of-concept demonstration. *Lancet.* 2017 May 6;389(10081):1821-30.

[16] Ramsey, N. F., Salari, E., Aarnoutse, E. J., Vansteensel, M. J., Bleichner, M. G. and Freudenburg, Z. V. Decoding spoken phones from sensorimotor cortex with high-density ECoG grids. *Neuroimage.* 2017 Oct 7. pii: S1053-8119(17)30824-8.

[17] Hamilton, L. S., Edwards, E. and Chang, E. F.. A Spatial Map of Onset and Sustained Responses to Speech in the Human Superior Temporal Gyrus. *Curr Biol.* 2018 Jun 18;28(12):1860-1871.

[18] Gearing, M. and Kennedy, P. R. Histological confirmation of myelinated neural filaments within the tip of the Neurotrophic Electrode after a decade of neural recordings. Accepted for publication by Frontiers.

[19] Lawhern, V., Solon, A., Waytowich, N., Gordon, S. M., Hung, C., and Lance, B. J. EEGNet: a compact convolutional neural network for EEG-based brain--computer interfaces. *J Neural Eng.* 2018: 22(1741-2552).

[20] Korik, A., Sosnik, R., Siddique, N. and Coyle, D. Decoding Imagined 3D Hand Movement Trajectories From EEG: Evidence to Support the Use of Mu, Beta, and Low Gamma Oscillations. *Front Neurosci.* 2018 20;12:130.

[21] Kennedy P.R., Dinal S. Andreasen, Jess Bartels, Princewill Ehirim, E. Joe Wright, Steven Seibert, Andre Joel Cervantes Validation of Neurotrophic Electrode long-term recordings in human cortex. Handbook of Biomedical Engineering. 2017.

[22] Kennedy P.R., Gambrell C, Ehirim P, and Cervantes A. Advances in the development of a speech prosthesis. Book chapter in Brain-Machine Interfaces: Uses and Developments accepted 2017.

ABOUT THE AUTHOR

Philip R. Kennedy, MD, PhD
CEO, Neural Signals Inc.

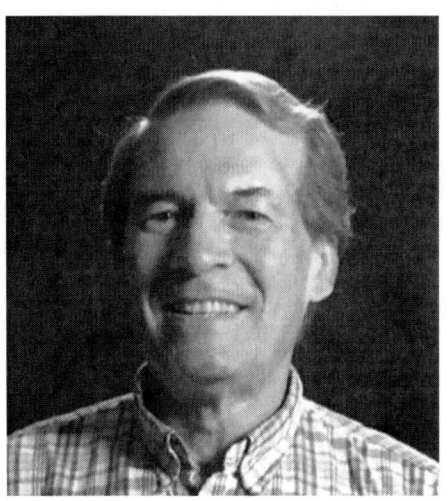

Phil Kennedy, MD, PhD, works as a neuroscientist and neurologist. He is chief scientist and CEO of Neural Signals Inc which he founded in 1989. The company is the leader in the field of Brain to Machine Interfacing. He has been developing and implanting the neurotrophic electrode since 1986 for long term recording of brain signals. Brain implantation has been performed in four locked-in subjects with a view to providing *communication via a computer*. He has implanted another subject in an attempt to *restore speech* and in 2014 he had himself implanted. His work has been published in major scientific journals and has been funded by the NIH and other agencies. He also has a part time neurology practice.

Publications:

2051
A Science Prediction story
Published on Kindle

Get a move on, Neuron!
A children's book available from the author's research laboratory at Neural Signals.com.

INDEX

A

academic success, 175
advancement, 200
age, 6, 8, 74, 80, 176
agencies, 195, 210
AI computer support, xvii
ALS, xviii, xix, 16, 87, 88, 92, 94, 125, 147, 149, 170, 181, 187, 189, 194
amine, 28
amyotrophic lateral sclerosis, 170
anatomy, 179
artificial intelligence, 11, 167
auditory cortex, 122
autonomic nervous system, xvi

B

bandwidth, 64
basic research, 165
Belize, v, xv, 53, 55, 57, 65, 127, 153, 154, 155, 156, 157, 159, 202
benefits, 154, 174, 195, 196, 202
bionic implants', xiv
blood, xvi, 17, 23, 30, 61, 90, 95, 123, 145
blood clot, 23
blood flow, 145
blood pressure, xvi, 17, 30, 61, 95, 123
blood vessels, 90, 95
blueprint, 39
bottom-up, 162
brain activity, 10, 17, 24, 111, 169, 181
brain functions, 12, 13, 154, 169
Brain Gate Project', xiv
brain-machine interface, xiv, 161, 167, 169, 170, 172, 174
brainstem, xvi, xvii, xx, 59, 61, 87, 89, 95, 117, 148, 184
brainstem stroke, xvii, xx, 59, 87, 89, 95, 117, 148, 184
breakdown, 60, 66, 93
brothers, 19, 29, 33, 66, 69, 70, 81
building blocks, 4, 9, 23, 111, 131

C

caffeine, 174
calibration, 92
cancer, 74, 189
candidates, 41, 57, 157
central nervous system, 6, 144, 205

challenges, 29, 33, 35, 52, 55, 165, 170, 171, 172
checks and balances, 177
children, 50, 62, 74, 88, 210
classification, 136
cognitive dysfunction, 16
cognitive function, 16
collaboration, 173
communication, xvii, xviii, 3, 5, 9, 29, 41, 46, 57, 66, 88, 89, 93, 170, 179, 180, 181, 182, 188, 189, 192, 193, 196, 210
communication system, xvii, 5, 88, 89, 179, 182, 188, 189
communication systems, 182
compilation, 169
complications, 60, 66, 127, 159, 187
comprehension, 128
computer, xvii, xviii, xix, 6, 10, 15, 21, 25, 29, 30, 34, 41, 47, 58, 63, 65, 88, 92, 93, 106, 109, 112, 118, 127, 143, 148, 149, 161, 166, 167, 170, 171, 178, 181, 182, 190, 193, 195, 196, 205, 207, 210
computer-controlled voice-generation device, xviii
computers, xiv, 23, 113, 136, 142, 144
conditioning, 56, 63, 91, 109, 123, 145
conscious knowledge, 39
consciousness, 39, 45, 53
continuous data, 23, 107
correlation coefficient, 136
correlations, 91, 137, 138, 162
cortex, xiii, 25, 40, 56, 90, 92, 93, 101, 102, 109, 122, 125, 127, 128, 129, 148, 150, 161, 162, 179, 205, 206, 207
cost, 57, 78, 142, 150, 191
craniotomy, xv, 102

D

data analysis, 25, 175
decision-making process, 156

decoding, 16, 17, 23, 30, 42, 55, 57, 58, 107, 111, 112, 131, 136, 138, 141, 145, 166, 167, 183, 205
deep brain stimulation, 174
Deep Brain Stimulation, xvi
deep learning, 11, 58, 136, 144
depth, 102, 157, 202, 205
disabilities, xiv, 178, 179, 193, 200
disappointment, 47
discriminant analysis, 206
disorder, 168, 194
dissociation, 162
doctors, 60, 61, 77
dominance, 40
dream, 159, 169

E

edema, 56
electrical fields, 54, 165
electrodes, x, xiii, xv, xix, 19, 22, 26, 54, 56, 57, 63, 89, 90, 91, 98, 103, 125, 127, 128, 130, 131, 139, 141, 142, 143, 144, 146, 149, 156, 157, 159, 170, 171, 177, 180, 181, 191, 192, 193, 195
electroencephalogram, 24
electroencephalography, 165
electron microscopy, 90
emotional intelligence, 45
emotional state, 174, 206
encouragement, xxii, 6
endurance, 11, 28, 143
energy, 8, 35, 47, 56, 157, 171
engineering, xiv, 167, 170, 195, 198
environment, xxii, 45, 148, 200
environmental control, 149, 178, 179, 188
epilepsy, 165, 194, 196
equipment, vi, 10, 11, 12, 16, 17, 21, 23, 24, 25, 30, 34, 35, 42, 169, 171, 173
essential tremor, 194
ethical issues, 172, 176

ethics, 172, 174, 195, 200, 202
evidence, 7, 123, 144, 145, 146, 162
evolution, v, xiv
execution, 163
exercises, 30, 56, 75
exoskeleton, 148
eye movement, xx, 67, 73

F

facial muscles, 130
faith, xv, 5, 48, 191
families, 60, 173, 174, 194
family members, 30, 173
fast processes, 171
fear, 26, 43
feelings, xvii, xxiii, 45, 47
fidelity, 171
financial, 189
fires, 45
flexibility, 92
flight, 3, 27, 33
food, 53, 62, 66, 77, 81, 187
football, 18, 46, 66, 165
formation, 13, 95, 143
foundations, 169
functional MRI, 101, 102, 190
funding, v, 57, 166, 175, 191, 199, 200

G

gay marriage, 43
Georgia, xix, xx, 6, 9, 21, 25, 40, 41, 88, 89, 90, 178, 185, 188, 189, 200
glasses, 29, 188
globalization, 51
glue, 28, 97, 106, 145
God, 157, 159, 201
governments, 150
grants, 67
growth, 40, 54, 57, 143, 183

guessing, 73
guidance, 173

H

hair, xv, 69, 72, 166
hallucinations, 88
handicapped people, 148
Hawking, Stephen, xviii, xix, 3, 4, 5, 6, 8, 16, 88
headache, 89
health, 29, 57, 58, 155, 177, 178
health effects, 178
heart rhythm, xvi
hemorrhage, 173
high school, 27, 72
history, 50, 109, 114, 159, 183, 199
human, v, xiii, xv, xvii, xix, xxii, xxiii, 3, 8, 9, 12, 15, 16, 18, 29, 31, 39, 41, 42, 48, 49, 54, 57, 91, 93, 127, 156, 159, 167, 168, 171, 176, 178, 191, 194, 195, 199, 200, 201, 202, 205, 206
human body, xvii, 9
human brain, v, xiii, 12, 39, 57, 168, 200, 206
human subjects, xv, 54, 91, 156, 194

I

identification, 112
iHuman, xiv
imagery, 163, 179, 181, 184, 200
images, 67, 148, 163, 180
imagination, 3, 4, 150
implant, x, xv, 16, 25, 29, 40, 41, 54, 55, 56, 63, 64, 90, 91, 93, 98, 101, 125, 127, 141, 142, 150, 171, 172, 175, 179, 184, 186, 187, 189, 190, 191, 195
impotence, xv
improvements, 34, 93, 165, 178
indigenous peoples, 50

individuals, xix, xxiii, 3, 4, 5, 6, 29, 34, 40, 42, 43, 49, 50, 52, 55, 57, 58, 174, 176
induction, 35, 98, 102, 103, 106
infection, 23, 98, 142, 159, 171
informed consent, 196
injury, xvii, 94, 165
insomnia, 157
intensive care unit, 6
interface, v, xiv, 11, 15, 29, 34, 36, 40, 91, 161, 165, 167, 169, 170, 171, 172, 174, 181, 182, 195, 206
interference, 42
interneurons, 161
intervention, xvii, 7
Ireland, v, 39, 43, 97, 198, 199, 201
issues, 62, 88, 89, 161, 176, 177

J

Jamestown, 81
joints, 148

K

kicks, 45

L

landscape, 29, 40, 175
languages, 4
lead, 27, 46, 92, 103, 151, 176, 191
learning, 13, 18, 50, 93, 121, 122, 136, 163, 165, 168, 183, 186
left hemisphere, 195
lifetime, 89, 90, 91, 97, 98, 143, 145, 170
light, xxv, 5, 8, 19, 47, 90, 117, 119, 130, 145, 154, 160
locked-in syndrome, xvii, xix, xxiii, 4, 7, 15, 34, 87
love, xxii, xxiii, 28, 47, 115, 136

lying, 5, 187

M

machine learning, v, 167, 168, 183
magnetic field, 165
magnetic fields, 165
mapping, 28, 57, 190
massive stroke, xvii
mathematics, xiv
matter, xxii, 46, 52, 53, 64, 75, 199
medical, vi, xv, 4, 5, 6, 7, 8, 12, 39, 46, 55, 61, 76, 157, 168, 169, 175, 177, 183, 187, 191, 200
medication, xv, 30, 128
medicine, 58, 153
memory, 19, 49, 88
mentor, v, 154, 155, 156, 159
methyl methacrylate, 97
Mexico, 127, 153, 154
microelectronics, 166
miniaturization, 150
misunderstanding, xxiii
models, 78, 161, 167, 176
modern science, 191, 201
monkey implants, xix
monkeys, xix, xx, 54, 89, 90, 91, 109, 127, 160, 161
motor behavior, 163
motor cortex, xiii, 40, 56, 90, 92, 93, 101, 102, 109, 122, 125, 127, 128, 129, 161, 162, 179, 206
motor neurons, 87, 157
motor task, 163
movement disorders, xvi
multisystem atrophy, xvi
muscles, xiv, 4, 7, 27, 89, 129, 161, 162, 167, 169, 170, 184, 186, 187, 206
music, 28, 36, 52, 63, 71, 117, 119, 121, 149
Musk, Elon, xv, 143, 166, 199, 200

Index

myopathy, 94, 186

N

nerve, xix, 88, 89, 90, 109, 121, 171, 177
nervous system, xvi, 168
Neural Interface Ecosystem, xiv
neural interfaces, xiv, xv, xvi, 166, 168, 195
neural network, v, 161, 163, 167, 168, 207
neural signals, xix, 10, 17, 21, 25, 28, 42, 57, 58, 90, 92, 94, 98, 106, 121, 128, 143, 145, 146, 150, 159, 167, 192, 206
neuralink, xv, 143, 166
neurites, xix, 40, 54, 68, 89, 90, 98, 106, 205
neuroimaging, 190
neurology, v, xiv, 154, 155, 159, 168, 169, 194, 210
neurons, v, xix, 13, 89, 90, 93, 98, 122, 143, 145, 161, 162, 163, 173, 175, 193
neuropathy, 148
neurophysiology, xiv
neuropsychiatry, v, 159
neuroscience, v, 39, 159, 166, 167, 168, 190
neuroscientist, v, xx, 10, 53, 155, 159, 167, 198, 199, 209
neurosurgery, v, xiv, 64, 97, 153, 154, 155, 157, 159, 190
nurses, 30
nursing care, 189
nursing home, 74, 75, 82
nutrients, 30, 35
nutrition, 95

O

occupational therapy, 75
operant conditioning, 161
opportunities, 165, 200
oral surgeon, 202
oral tradition, 50

organ, 194
outpatients, 56
outreach, 195
ownership, 55

P

pain, xvi, 12, 28, 41, 42, 46, 62, 64, 128, 179, 187
paralysis, xvii, 4, 6, 15, 40, 41, 54, 56, 87, 148, 164
parents, 28, 64, 68, 79, 95, 98, 150, 189
participants, 46, 173, 181
pathways, 40, 54, 95
permission, iv, 39, 54, 91
personality traits, 13
pharmaceuticals, xiv
pharmacology, 168
physical interaction, 31
physical therapist, 7, 75, 80
playing, 55, 70
pneumonia, xviii, 6, 61, 73, 80, 189
police, 81, 150, 181
population, 163
problem-solver, 30
professionals, 156
project, xv, xx, 21, 35, 57, 64, 142, 181, 183, 184
prostheses, v, 122, 162
prosthesis, xiii, 58, 125
prosthetic device, 90, 91
psychopharmacology, 190

Q

quality of life, 46, 57, 88, 156, 194, 195
quarterback, 69

R

radar, 70, 157
radio, 42, 171, 179
reading, xiv, xxv, 89, 174, 194, 195, 202
real time, 9, 11, 17, 21, 23, 31, 34, 45, 50, 52, 161
reality, 13, 19, 31, 42, 53, 165, 170
recognition, 17, 166, 177
recommendations, iv
recovery, 7, 23, 24, 25, 28, 56, 57, 64, 189
recovery process, 56
redundancy, 163
rehabilitation, 56, 74, 178
repair, 12, 28, 95, 147
repetitions, 122, 137
requirements, 177, 191
researchers, 6, 41, 109, 128, 172, 173, 174, 176, 177, 178, 183
resolution, 93, 144, 145
response, 17, 31, 36, 124, 179, 181
right hemisphere, 195
risk, v, xv, 55, 93, 126, 167, 177, 178, 195
risks, 173, 174, 175, 177, 191, 195, 196
robot, xv, 180, 182
robotic arms, xiv, 91
routines, 29, 33, 46
rugby, 69
rules, 18, 79, 191

S

school, 12, 39, 61, 66, 71, 72, 80
sciatic nerve, xix, 89, 90
science, xvi, xviii, xxiii, 8, 19, 25, 35, 40, 53, 58, 89, 147, 167, 176, 178, 191, 196, 201
self-image, 49
seller, 142
sensory modalities, 163
short-term memory, 161
signals, xiv, xix, xxi, 10, 16, 17, 21, 25, 28, 35, 40, 41, 42, 54, 55, 57, 58, 62, 67, 89, 90, 91, 92, 93, 94, 97, 98, 106, 121, 125, 128, 141, 143, 144, 145, 146, 148, 149, 150, 159, 167, 169, 170, 171, 172, 173, 174, 181, 183, 192, 193, 206, 209
Silicon Valley, 200
skin, 66, 170, 171, 179, 181, 187, 188, 191
skin cancer, 188
society, 151, 154, 155
software, 11, 16, 25, 30, 34, 40, 65, 107, 109, 115, 142, 166, 178, 206
solution, xix, 40, 89, 102, 141, 142, 154, 173, 176
speech generation, 10
speech processing, 54
spelling, 144, 181, 182, 186, 189
spinal cord, xvii, 6, 87, 88, 147, 148, 156, 161, 165
spinal cord injury, xvii, 165
state, 5, 15, 16, 57, 87, 173, 175, 192, 198
stimulation, xvi, 12, 89, 148, 161, 163, 206
stroke, xvii, xx, 7, 22, 41, 59, 61, 62, 87, 89, 95, 117, 123, 148, 165, 170, 173, 178, 184
structure, 24, 101, 167, 168
survival, xix, 58, 164
symptoms, xvi, 194
syndrome, xvii, xix, xxiii, 4, 7, 15, 34, 87, 194
synthesis, 6, 146, 168

T

target, 35, 101, 102, 116, 136, 137, 161
teachers, 71, 72
techniques, xiv, 165, 167, 173, 179, 182, 189, 190
technologies, xiv, 41, 164, 165, 168, 179, 182

technology, v, 6, 23, 50, 148, 150, 167, 171, 173, 174, 175, 183, 191, 196, 200, 202
teenage girls, 18
temperature, 165
testing, 11, 40, 41, 57, 176
tetraplegics, xiv
therapist, xvii, 4, 9, 72, 73, 75
therapy, vi, 9, 18, 30, 56, 75, 169, 196
thoughts, xvii, 21, 23, 41, 42, 45, 47, 50, 166, 168, 169, 199
tissue, 40, 68, 90, 91, 97, 103, 143, 145
tracks, v, 4, 6, 29, 198, 199, 200
training, 30, 66, 116, 144, 154, 156, 168, 169, 184, 189, 194
trajectory, 166
transformation, 23, 48
treatment, xiv, xv, 61, 169, 174, 177

U

universe, v, 8, 47, 157, 159
Utah array, xiii, xix, 65, 143

V

variables, 163
variations, 176

vector, 206
victims, xvii, 3, 49
visualization, 179

W

water, 18, 24, 36, 75, 106
weakness, 128, 177
well-being, 58, 177
wheelchairs, xiv, 77, 81, 148, 179
wireless devices, 101, 128, 141
wires, xix, 26, 65, 68, 90, 92, 97, 98, 103, 125, 127, 131, 141, 145, 191
word format, 57
working memory, 190
worldwide, 148
wrestling, 18, 29, 70

X

X-axis, 112, 114

Y

Y-axis, 112, 114